QUESTIONS AND ANSWERS IN NEURO-OPHTHALMOLOGY

A Case-Based Approach

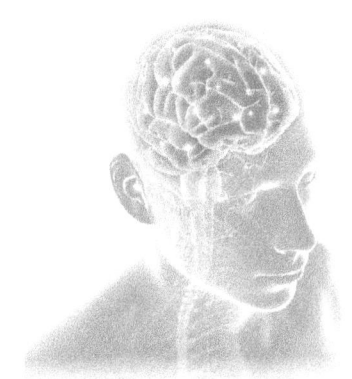

QUESTIONS AND ANSWERS IN NEURO-OPHTHALMOLOGY

A Case-Based Approach

Andrew G. Lee MD

Houston Methodist Hospital, Houston, TX, USA
Chair, Department of Ophthalmology

Professor of Ophthalmology, Neurology and Neurosurgery
Weill Cornell Medical College, New York City, NY, USA

Clinical Professor of Ophthalmology: The University of Texas Medical Branch (UTMB)
at Galveston, TX and the UT MD Anderson Cancer Center, Houston, TX, USA

Adjunct Professor, Ophthalmology: Baylor College of Medicine and the
University of Iowa Hospitals and Clinics, Iowa City, IA, USA

Nagham Al Zubidi MD & Arielle Spitze MD

Department of Ophthalmology, Neuro-ophthalmology Section,
Houston Methodist Hospital

Sushma Yalamanchili MD

Methodist Eye Associates
Houston Methodist Hospital

Assistant Professor of Ophthalmology
Weill Cornell Medical College

Adjunct Assistant Professor
Department of Ophthalmology and Visual Science
The University of Texas Medical Branch (UTMB) at Galveston

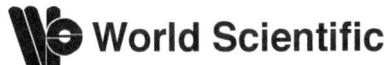

World Scientific

NEW JERSEY · LONDON · SINGAPORE · BEIJING · SHANGHAI · HONG KONG · TAIPEI · CHENNAI

Published by

World Scientific Publishing Co. Pte. Ltd.

5 Toh Tuck Link, Singapore 596224

USA office: 27 Warren Street, Suite 401-402, Hackensack, NJ 07601

UK office: 57 Shelton Street, Covent Garden, London WC2H 9HE

Library of Congress Cataloging-in-Publication Data
Lee, Andrew G., author.
 Questions and answers in neuro-ophthalmology : a case-based approach / Andrew G. Lee, Nagham Al Zubidi, Arielle Spitze.
   p. ; cm.
 Includes bibliographical references.
 ISBN 978-9814578769 (hardcover : alk. paper) -- ISBN 978-9814578776 (pbk. : alk. paper)
 I. Al Zubidi, Nagham, author. II. Spitze, Arielle, author. III. Title.
 [DNLM: 1. Cranial Nerve Diseases--Case Reports. 2. Cranial Nerve Diseases--Problems and Exercises. 3. Eye Diseases--Case Reports. 4. Eye Diseases--Problems and Exercises. 5. Eye Manifestations--Case Reports. 6. Eye Manifestations--Problems and Exercises. 7. Neurologic Manifestations--Case Reports. 8. Neurologic Manifestations--Problems and Exercises. WW 18.2]
 RE49
 617.70076--dc23

                                          2013046933

British Library Cataloguing-in-Publication Data
A catalogue record for this book is available from the British Library.

Contents

Contents

Acknowledgments

Dr. Lee would like to recognize the critical importance of his current and former residents and fellows in conceiving the core idea for this book and for providing the basis for many of the commonly asked questions in neuro-ophthalmology which might be of additional interest to a general ophthalmologist. He also wishes to acknowledge the crucial role of his brother, Richard Lee, in both inspiring and challenging him with his intellectual curiosity and his inquisitive mind and who has been a lifelong source of academic and personal guidance and motivation. In addition, Dr. Lee wishes to give thanks to his professional colleagues, Dr. Neil Miller (Johns Hopkins Hospital), Dr. Tony Arnold (UCLA), and Dr. Paul Brazis (Mayo Clinic), for their wisdom, mentorship, and friendship; to his sister, Amy Lee Wirts MD, for being an equally important and inspirational source of deeper and metaphysical life questions; to his parents, Alberto C. Lee MD and Rosalind L. Go Lee MD, for instilling the tenets of science and medicine in him and for their years of love and support; to his wife, Hilary A. Beaver MD, for her eternal love, companionship, friendship, and patience through the work of nine medical textbooks and 350 papers; and to his children, Rachael E. Lee (aged 11) and Virginia A. Lee (aged 9), whom he hopes will one day assume the mantle of three generations of physicians in the Lee and Beaver families.

Disclaimer

Although Andrew Lee MD is a member of the Ophthalmology Residency Review Committee (RRC), an examiner for the oral board examination of the American Board of Ophthalmology (ABO), and a question writer for the Ophthalmic Knowledge and Assessment Program (OKAP), the questions and answers in this textbook are not designed for the ABO or other board review purposes. The content of the book is the work of the authors alone, who take sole responsibility for the work, and the content does not represent or reflect the views of the RRC, ABO, or OKAP in any way.

Introduction

This book is designed to answer the routine and common questions of medical students, residents, fellows, and general ophthalmologists about garden-variety topics in neuro-ophthalmology. It is not intended to be all-inclusive or comprehensive and instead is meant to challenge readers to consider the distinctive symptoms, differentiating signs, and distinguishing radiographic or laboratory features of common neuro-ophthalmic problems. Other reference sources can provide more in-depth analysis or detail for anatomy, pathogenesis, or other basic science content for these conditions. Our intention is simply to provide a starting point for clinicians interested in the key clinical history, examination, laboratory, or radiographic findings in these common neuro-ophthalmic presentations. We hope that you will take the opportunity to write and answer your own questions for these and other topics as the process itself of reading and writing questions is an additional mechanism to leverage your lifelong learning in neuro-ophthalmology.

1

Anisocoria — Abnormally Small Pupil (Horner Syndrome)

Arielle Spitze MD, Diana Chao MD, Nagham Al-Zubidi MD, Sushma Yalamanchili MD, and Andrew G. Lee MD

CASE

A 46-year-old man presented with a two-week history of acute-onset left upper eyelid drooping. He also had left eye, ear, and neck pain, as well as numbness and pain along his left cheek. He denied trauma and was not taking any medications or eye drops. The remainder of his medical and ocular history was unremarkable. Best-corrected visual acuity was 20/20 in both eyes (OU). External exam showed left upper eyelid ptosis of 2 mm. There was no upside-down ptosis. In the dark, his right pupil measured 6 mm and his left pupil measured 4 mm with a dilation lag in the left eye (OS) with the lights dimmed. In the light, the right pupil measured 3 mm and the left pupil measured 1.5 mm (see Fig. 1.1). There was no relative afferent pupillary defect or light-near dissociation. Extraocular motility, intraocular pressure measurements, and slit lamp examination were normal OU. One drop of topical apraclonidine 0.5% was administered OU. After 30 minutes, the left ptosis improved, and the previously larger right pupil was now smaller and the previously smaller left pupil was now larger (see Fig. 1.2). Dilated fundus exam was normal OU. Corneal sensation and facial sensation in the V_1 and V_2 distributions were normal. Magnetic resonance imaging (MRI) of the face, orbits, head, and neck down to the level of the second thoracic vertebra revealed

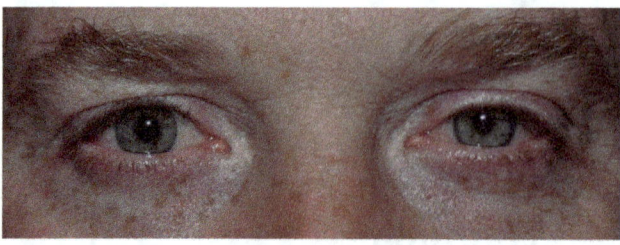

Fig. 1.1. External photo demonstrating left ptosis and left miosis. The anisocoria was worse in the dark as compared to the light.

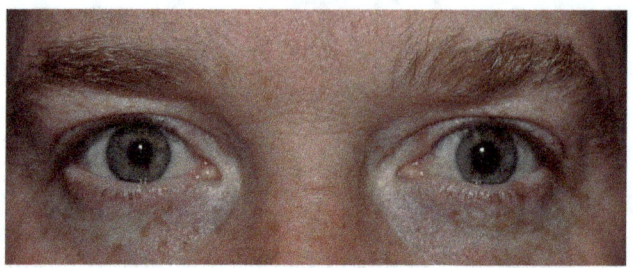

Fig. 1.2. External photo illustrating the reversal of anisocoria and mild lid retraction after apraclonidine administration.

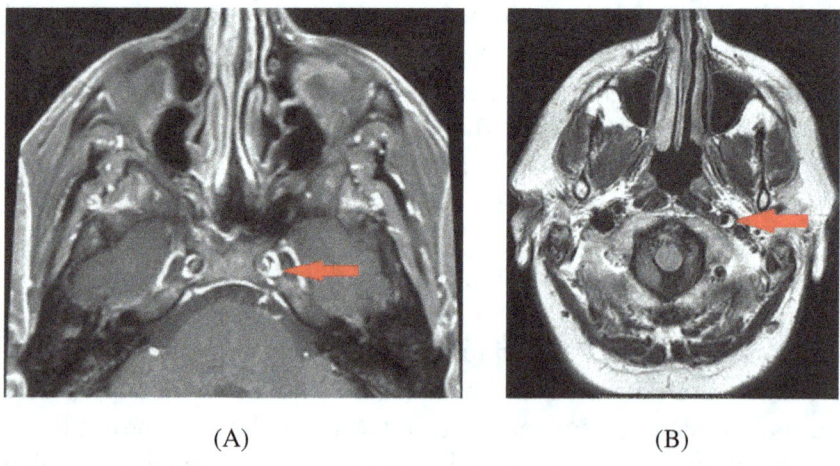

(A) (B)

Fig. 1.3. (A) T1 post-gadolinium MRI with fat suppression showing the crescent sign of the left internal carotid artery flow void. A similar finding is seen in (B) on MRI T2 axial FLAIR.

hyperintense signal intensity in the wall of the distal left internal carotid artery (i.e., the crescent sign) consistent with a left carotid dissection (see Fig. 1.3). Magnetic resonance angiogram (MRA) of the head and neck confirmed a dissection of the distal left cervical internal carotid artery (ICA) (see Fig. 1.4).

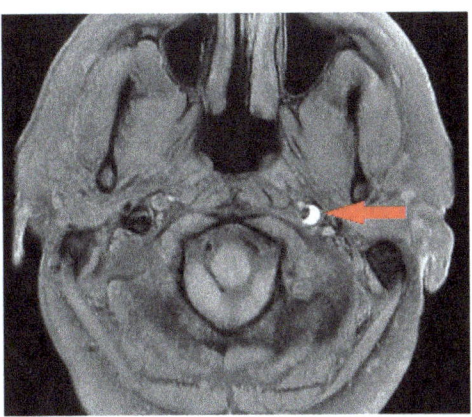

Fig. 1.4. MRA demonstrating the crescent-shaped area of increased signal along the left side of the left internal carotid artery beginning at the level just above the odontoid process and extending up to the level just below the skull base, consistent with a dissection. The left internal carotid artery is also narrowed by approximately 30% in this region.

Question 1	Question 2
Which of the following findings is most likely due to an internal carotid artery dissection?	**Which of the following signs is most consistent with Horner syndrome?**
A. Ipsilateral complete ptosis B. Contralateral monocular visual loss C. Contralateral upper extremity weakness D. Ipsilateral pupillary mydriasis	A. Hyperhidrosis of the face B. Anhidrosis of the face C. Pupillary mydriasis and anisocoria D. Relative afferent pupillary defect

Question 3	Question 4
Which of the following is the most likely location of a lesion in a patient with Horner syndrome?	Which of the following pharmacologic tests would confirm Horner syndrome?
A. Sympathetic pathway B. Parasympathetic pathway C. Both autonomic pathways D. Neither autonomic pathway	A. 1% pilocarpine B. 1% apraclonidine C. 0.1% pilocarpine D. 1% homatropine
Question 5	Question 6
Which of the following is most consistent with a positive topical cocaine test in Horner syndrome?	Which of the following results of topical apraclonidine testing is most consistent with Horner syndrome?
A. Both pupils dilate B. Both pupils constrict C. The smaller pupil will dilate to a lesser degree than the normal pupil D. Reversal of the anisocoria such that the smaller pupil will be more dilated than the normal pupil	A. Both pupils dilate B. Both pupils constrict C. Smaller pupil constricts D. Reversal of anisocoria
Question 7	Question 8
Which of the following is the mechanism for a positive apraclonidine test in Horner syndrome?	Which of the following is the localization of a right Horner syndrome if there is poor dilation OD and normal dilation OS after topical hydroxyamphetamine?
A. Aberrant regeneration B. Adrenergic supersensitivity C. Cholinergic denervation D. Cholinergic supersensitivity	A. Preganglionic, second-order neuron B. Preganglionic, central neuron C. Neuromuscular junction D. Postganglionic, third-order neuron

Question 9	Question 10
Which of the following is the best imaging study for an acute painful Horner syndrome?	Which of the following is the characteristic radiographic sign for carotid artery dissection?
A. Cranial MRI and MRA down to T2 in the chest **B.** MRI and MRA of the head and neck **C.** MRI of the brain with MRA of circle of Willis **D.** MRI of the brain and orbit with gadolinium	**A.** Full moon sign of isointensity **B.** Solar sign of hypointensity **C.** Crescent sign of hyperintensity **D.** Dilated superior ophthalmic vein

EXPLANATIONS

The solution to Question 1 is C.

The most common presenting symptom of ICA dissection is ipsilateral headache or neck pain, while the most common sign is an ipsilateral Horner syndrome (HS). HS can be present in up to 58% of ICA dissections and contralateral neurologic deficits (e.g., hemiparesis, hemisensory loss, or homonymous hemianopsia) may occur due to ipsilateral thromboembolic hemispheric carotid ischemic dysfunction.[1–4] Ipsilateral monocular visual loss can also occur with carotid dissection from branch or central retinal artery thromboembolic disease. Dysgeusia (distortion of the sense of taste) can also occur in patients with a carotid dissection. Occasionally, these neurologic symptoms may be delayed for weeks to months following the initial dissection as the thrombosis propagates.[5] The neurologic signs and symptoms may be transient (i.e., transient ischemic attacks including amaurosis fugax) or permanent (i.e., ischemic infarction). Mild ipsilateral ptosis and miosis with anisocoria greater in the dark are the hallmarks of HS. Complete ptosis, however, does not occur because in HS there is denervation of the involved oculosympathetically innervated muscle in the upper lid (i.e., the Müller muscle) as well as involvement of the equivalent but unnamed sympathetic muscle in the lower lid (i.e., upside-down ptosis). This ptosis related to HS can only produce one or two millimeters of ptosis (upper lid involvement) (see Figs. 1.1 and 1.2) and not a complete ptosis. This is in contrast to third nerve palsy-related denervation of the levator palpebrae superioris, which can produce a partial or complete ipsilateral ptosis. In addition, HS produces pupillary miosis and not mydriasis.

The solution to Question 2 is B.

As noted above, the classic triad of HS includes ipsilateral mild ptosis or upside-down ptosis, miosis, and facial or body (central HS) anhidrosis. HS can result from a lesion anywhere in the ipsilateral oculosympathetic pathway.[6] In HS, the lesion occurs along the sympathetic pathway, so the upper eyelid ptosis is due to the paresis of the Müller muscle and the upside-down ptosis occurs from involvement of the lower lid sympathetically innervated retractor. The ipsilateral miosis is caused by paresis of the iris dilator muscle. The anisocoria is greater in the dark because of poor or no dilation from the oculosympathetic paresis. Because the sweat glands are also sympathetically innervated, anhidrosis occurs in HS as well. First-order (central) lesions can produce ipsilateral body anhidrosis, and second-order neuron lesions can cause anhidrosis of the ipsilateral face. Third-order neuron lesions may result in anhidrosis of the forehead only (V_1). Hyperhidrosis can occur in patients with systemic autonomic dysfunction affecting both parasympathetic and sympathetic innervation.[7] In the presence of a parasympathetic (rather than sympathetic denervation–related HS) pupil dysfunction (e.g., Adie's tonic pupil), segmental systemic hyperhidrosis and anhidrosis might represent the generalized autonomic neuropathy of Ross syndrome.[8]

The solution to Question 3 is A.

The oculosympathetic disruption in this case was due to a dissection of the left internal carotid artery, affecting sympathetic fibers traveling in proximity to the arterial wall (shown in Figs. 1.3 and 1.4). The ocular sympathetic nervous system fibers originate in the posterior hypothalamus and travel down the brainstem and spinal cord to synapse in the ciliospinal nucleus of Budge–Waller (C8–T2). The second-order neuron then ascends via the cervical sympathetic chain, over the apex of the lung (where it might be affected by the apical Pancoast tumor), and synapses at the superior cervical ganglion (at the level of the carotid artery bifurcation (C2) and the angle of the jaw). The third-order neuron continues in the wall of the bifurcated carotid artery. The sympathetic fibers destined for the pupil ascend intracranially with the internal carotid artery and join for a short course with cranial nerve (CN) VI in the cavernous sinus. The sympathetic fibers then join the nasociliary branch of V_1, and enter the orbit via the long ciliary nerve to innervate the Müller muscle of the lid and the iris dilator muscle. In contrast, the oculomotor nerve (i.e., third cranial nerve) carries the parasympathetic innervation to the sphincter of the pupil. A lesion in the parasympathetic pathway would produce a dilated and poorly reactive pupil rather than HS. Lesions of the cavernous sinus can affect both the sympathetic (HS) and parasympathetic (third nerve) pathways of the pupil.

The solution to Question 4 is B.

The most appropriate initial pharmacologic testing for a patient with suspected HS is to use topical 0.5–1% apraclonidine[9] or 4–10% cocaine.[10] In contrast, topical pilocarpine is used to test parasympathetic dysfunction. Dilute, low-dose (0.1%) pilocarpine is used for denervation supersensitivity in Adie's tonic pupil and 1% pilocarpine for pharmacologically blocked dilated pupils. Topical epinephrine is a direct-acting sympathomimetic and will dilate the pupil even in an eye affected with HS. In fact, epinephrine can dilate the involved pupil to a greater extent than the fellow (control) normal eye. However, the test is not sufficiently sensitive or specific to diagnose HS as compared with topical apraclonidine or topical cocaine testing. Homatropine is a parasympatholytic and will dilate the pupil in both a normal eye and an eye affected with HS.

The solution to Question 5 is C.

When using 4–10% cocaine to test a patient with suspected HS, a positive result is a post cocaine anisocoria of 0.8 mm or more, with the HS pupil likely being the smaller pupil.[10] Cocaine is an indirect sympathomimetic and blocks the re-uptake of norepinephrine at the neuromuscular junction. After topical cocaine is administered in the normal eye, the pupil will dilate because there is more norepinephrine at the neuromuscular junction to stimulate the iris dilator muscle. However, in HS, due to sympathetic denervation, there is little to no norepinephrine at the neuromuscular junction, so the pupil will dilate poorly, even with the cocaine. Normal pupils will dilate rather than constrict after the administration of cocaine. Parasympathomimetic agents (e.g., pilocarpine 1%) will constrict normal pupils. Reversal of the anisocoria (i.e., the smaller HS pupil dilates and the larger, normal pupil constricts slightly) is the positive endpoint for topical apraclonidine testing in HS.[9]

The solution to Question 6 is D.

A positive test result when using topical 0.5–1% apraclonidine in a patient with suspected HS is a reversal of the anisocoria.[9] Apraclonidine is an alpha-2 agonist and normally causes pupillary constriction in normal patients but the drug is also a weak alpha-1 agonist (which causes pupillary dilation). In a normal pupil (e.g., physiologic anisocoria), apraclonidine will cause pupillary constriction in both eyes because of the stronger alpha-2 action. However, in sympathetically denervated eyes (i.e., the HS pupil), the iris dilator muscle develops adrenergic supersensitivity, which allows the previously weaker alpha-1 agonist activity to predominate. This causes pupillary dilation in the denervated eye only. Thus, after instillation of apraclonidine, a positive result for HS is a reversal of anisocoria (the previously smaller pupil will be larger and the previously larger pupil will become smaller).

The solution to Question 7 is B.

The mechanism of a positive apraclonidine test for HS is alpha adrenergic supersensitivity of the iris dilator muscle.[9] Cholinergic denervation supersensitivity is the basis of the topical dilute pilocarpine 0.1% test in Adie's tonic pupil. Aberrant regeneration of fibers destined originally for the ciliary body that now innervate the pupil produces the finding of light-near dissociation in Adie's tonic pupil.

The solution to Question 8 is D.

After HS is confirmed with either topical cocaine or topical apra-clonidine, topical hydroxyamphetamine may be used to further localize the lesion to the preganglionic (first- or second-order neuron) or postganglionic neuron. Hydroxyamphetamine releases norepine-phrine from the presynaptic terminal, causing pupillary dilation in a normal eye. In a preganglionic HS lesion, the postganglionic neuron remains intact and therefore hydroxyamphetamine will dilate the affected HS pupil to the same degree as it dilates the normal pupil. However, in postganglionic HS (third-order neuron) the affected pupil does not dilate as well to hydroxyamphetamine.[11] Thus, in a postganglionic lesion, the degree of anisocoria will increase following hydroxyamphetamine administration. Although many textbooks still argue for pharmacologic localization with hydroxyamphetamine, the sensitivity and specificity of the test is not sufficient to completely obviate imaging of the entire oculosympathetic pathway in HS.[12] In addition, transsynaptic degeneration can produce false positive and false negative hydroxyamphetamine testing in children, diminishing the clinical application of this test. Neuromuscular pharmacologic blockade can cause a dilated or constricted pupil depending on the agent.[13]

The solution to Question 9 is A.

One imaging study protocol in the evaluation of HS is MRI and MRA of the brain, orbit, neck, and chest down to the level of thoracic level 2 (T2) with gadolinium and fat saturation (see Fig. 1.3). Because a lesion at any location along the oculosympathetic pathway may produce HS, it is crucial to image the entire pathway. In the acute setting where carotid dissection is the main concern, CT with CTA of the head and neck could be performed,[14] but if negative, other non-vascular etiologies have to be considered as the cause of Horner syndrome. Thus, contrast head and neck MRI and MRA imaging of the entire course of the oculosympathetic pathway might still be necessary.[15] MRI and/or MRA of the brain alone, the orbit alone, or the brain and orbit without the neck are insufficient for imaging the entirety of the oculosympathetic pathway. Contrast material increases the sensitivity and specificity of both MRI and CT but some patients (e.g., those with renal failure) may not be able to tolerate contrast material for either MRI or CT scanning. Fat saturation allows the normal fat signal on T1 to be suppressed and can allow visualization of lesions that might be obscured by fat, including acute hemorrhage.

The solution to Question 10 is C.

The characteristic and distinctive radiographic sign for carotid artery dissection is the crescent sign. This crescent of hyperintense signal on T1 represents the blood dissecting in the false lumen of the acute dissection[16] (see Figs. 1.3 and 1.4). While a dilated superior ophthalmic vein can be present in cases of increased cerebral venous pressure such as carotid-cavernous fistulas, it is not a characteristic sign of carotid artery dissection.

SUMMARY

The classic triad of Horner syndrome includes ipsilateral ptosis, miosis, and anhidrosis.[6] The ptosis is usually only a few millimeters rather than a more pronounced ptosis such as that seen in cranial nerve III palsy. This is due to a difference in affected muscles. Horner syndrome affects the sympathetically innervated Müller muscle, while cranial nerve III palsy affects the levator palpebrae superioris muscle. Horner syndrome is diagnosed on examination by first demonstrating that anisocoria is present and greater in the dark (showing the dysfunctional pupil is the smaller one). Sympathetic denervation can then be confirmed using either topical apraclonidine or cocaine testing.[9,10] The mechanism by which apraclonidine causes a reversal of anisocoria is via weak alpha-1 agonism and stronger alpha-2 agonism. Thus, apraclonidine will dilate a supersensitive sympathetically denervated pupil (Horner pupil) due to the weak alpha-1 agonism, and constrict a normal pupil due to the stronger alpha-2 agonism. If an acute Horner syndrome is present, topical testing might not be available in a timely manner and the imaging study of choice should evaluate the entire oculosympathetic pathway, which includes the head, neck, and upper chest down to the level of T2. MRI of the brain, orbits, and neck (down to T2) with and without gadolinium is the initial study of choice, followed by MRA of the head and neck to evaluate for life-threatening causes of Horner syndrome, specifically carotid dissection.[15] CT with CTA of the head and neck might be faster in the emergent setting especially when carotid dissection is the main consideration. After a positive topical apraclonidine or cocaine test for HS, topical hydroxyamphetamine is suggested for localization of the lesion to the pre- or postganglionic neuron[12] but the test is unfortunately neither 100% sensitive nor specific enough to completely obviate imaging in HS.

REFERENCES

1. Tobin J, Flitman S. (2008) Cluster-like headaches associated with internal carotid artery dissection responsive to verapamil. *Headache* **48**:461–466.
2. Bougousslavsky J, Despland PA, Regli F. (1987) Spontaneous carotid dissection with acute stroke. *Arch Neurol* **44**:137–140.
3. Divjak I, Slankamenac P, Jovicevic M, *et al.* (2011) A case series of 22 patients with internal carotid artery dissection. *Med Pregl* **64**:575–578.
4. Patel RR, Adam R, Maldjian C, *et al.* (2012) Cervical carotid artery dissection: current review of diagnosis and treatment. *Cardiol Rev* **20**:145–152.
5. Pozzati E, Giuliani G, Poppi M, Faenza A. (1989) Blunt traumatic carotid dissection with delayed symptoms. *Stroke* **20**:412–416.
6. Nagy AN, Hayman LA, Diaz-Marchan PJ, Lee AG. (1997) Horner's syndrome due to first-order neuron lesions of the oculosympathetic pathway. *AJR Am J Roentgenol* **169**:581–584.

7. Korpelainen JT, Sotaniemi KA, Myllyla VV. (1992) Hyperhidrosis as a reflection of autonomic failure in patients with acute hemispheral brain infarction. An evaporimetric study. *Stroke* **23**:1271–1275.

8. Hagemann G, Bartke T. (2006) Images in clinical medicine. Adie's pupil in the Ross syndrome. *N Engl J Med* **355**:e5.

9. Morales J, Brown SM, Abdul-Ralim AS, Crosson CE. (2000) Ocular effects of apraclonidine in Horner Syndrome. *Arch Ophthalmol* **118**:951–954.

10. Kardon RH, Denison CE, Brown CK, Thompson HS. (1990) Critical evaluation of the cocaine test in the diagnosis of Horner's syndrome. *Arch Ophthalmol* **108**:384–387.

11. Cremer SA, Thompson HS, Digre KB, Kardon RH. (1990) Hydroxyamphetamine mydriasis in Horner's syndrome. *Am J Ophthalmol* **110**:71–76.

12. Maloney WF, Young BR, Moyer NJ. (1980) Evaluation of the causes and accuracy of pharmacologic localization of Horner's syndrome. *Am J Ophthalmol* **90**:394–402.

13. Weinstein JM, Zweifel TJ, Thompson HS. (1980) Congenital Horner's syndrome. *Arch Ophthalmol* **98**:1074–1078.

14. Leclerc X, Godefroy O, Salhi A, *et al.* (1996) Helical CT for the diagnosis of extracranial internal carotid artery dissection. *Stroke* **27**:461–466.

15. Vertinsky AT, Schwartz NE, Fischbein NJ, *et al.* (2008) Comparison of multidetector CT angiography and MR imaging of cervical artery dissection. *AJNR Am J Neuroradiol* **29**:1753–1760.

16. Provenzale JM. (1995) Dissection of the internal carotid and vertebral arteries: imaging features. *AJR Am J Roentgenol* **5**:1099–1104.

2

Anisocoria — Abnormally Large Pupil

Arielle Spitze MD, Alexander S. Davis MD,
Nagham Al-Zubidi MD, Sushma Yalamanchili MD,
and Andrew G. Lee MD

CASE

A 60-year-old woman presented with a three-week history of a dilated right pupil associated with symptoms of difficulty reading, increased photosensitivity, and headache when going outside. Past medical history was significant for well-controlled hypertension on antihypertensive agents and stable mitral valve prolapse. Past ocular history was significant for recent blepharoplasty in both eyes (OU). The remainder of the medical, surgical, and social history was unremarkable. On examination, the patient had a distance visual acuity of 20/25 OU but decreased near vision of J16 in the right eye (OD) and J1 in the left eye (OS) with a correction of +2.50 sphere. Pupils measured 6.5 mm OD and 5 mm OS in the dark and 6 mm OD and 3 mm OS in the light. There was no relative afferent pupillary defect (RAPD). There was however mild light-near dissociation noted OD. Additionally, the right pupil had an ovoid shape, elongated vertically (Fig. 2.1). Motility examination was full OU and the patient was orthophoric in all diagnostic positions of gaze. Intraocular pressure measurements were 16 mmHg OU. Automated visual field testing (Humphrey 24-2) was normal OU. External exam was negative for ptosis, scalp tenderness, or temporal artery nodularity. On slit lamp examination, there was sectoral iris sphincter paresis (i.e., sectoral paresis) with constriction of only the non-paretic segments at near (vermiform movements of iris).

There were no iris transillumination defects, iris atrophy, anterior or posterior synechiae, or anterior chamber cells present. Topical dilute pilocarpine testing (0.1%) OU showed constriction of the right pupil but no change in the left pupil size (Fig. 2.2).

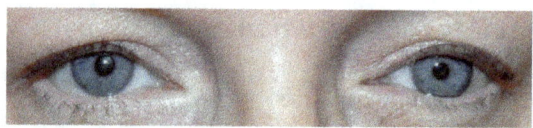

Fig. 2.1. External exam showing an irregular, larger, oval-shaped right pupil, demonstrating sectoral iris sphincter paresis.

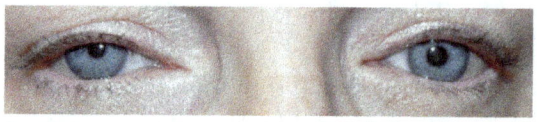

Fig. 2.2. External exam following dilute 0.1% pilocarpine testing, with constriction of the right pupil. Note that although the dilute pilocarpine was placed in both eyes, no constriction was seen in the left eye (normal pupil response to dilute pilocarpine).

Question 1	Question 2
Which of the following signs is the most likely presenting symptom of a patient with Adie's tonic pupil?	Which of the following signs is most likely in a typical chronic Adie's tonic pupil?
A. No symptoms **B.** Severe headache **C.** Ipsilateral ptosis **D.** Binocular diplopia	**A.** Normal pupillary reaction to light **B.** Ipsilateral or contralateral ptosis **C.** Segmental palsy of iris sphincter **D.** Lack of pupillary near reaction

Question 3	Question 4
Which of the following topical pharmacologic tests would be most diagnostic for an Adie's tonic pupil?	A patient presents with a dilated, irregular pupil OD six weeks following a red eye OD. There is no pupillary response to light, near stimuli, or dilute or normal-strength topical pilocarpine OD. The left pupil is normal. Which of the following is the most likely finding OD?
A. 1% pilocarpine **B.** 0.1% pilocarpine **C.** 1% apraclonidine **D.** 0.1% brimonidine	**A.** Light-near dissociation **B.** Segmental iris sphincter palsy **C.** Posterior synechiae **D.** Exotropia and hypotropia
Question 5	Question 6
A 30-year-old woman presents with a 6 mm dilated pupil OS and severe headache. In this patient, which of the following parts of the eye examination would be most diagnostic of a third nerve palsy as the etiology for the anisocoria?	A 15-year-old woman presents to the emergency room for evaluation of new-onset anisocoria for two days. In the light, her pupils measure 2 mm OD and 7 mm OS. The left pupil does not react to light or near stimuli. Slit lamp biomicroscopy, motility, and lid examinations are all normal. Her medical history is negative with the exception of surgery performed the day before for a broken ankle. Which of the following is the most likely diagnosis?
A. Extraocular motility **B.** Pupillary near response **C.** Relative afferent pupillary defect **D.** Topical pilocarpine	**A.** Cranial nerve III palsy **B.** Pharmacologic dilation **C.** Pupillary block glaucoma **D.** Benign episodic mydriasis

EXPLANATIONS

The solution to Question 1 is A.

Although photophobia (increased sensitivity to light) is a common presenting symptom for patients with a tonic pupil (including Adie's tonic pupil) and some patients report the anisocoria as their chief complaint, many patients are asymptomatic or have the anisocoria detected by family members or friends. Difficulty with near vision or reported blurry vision at near is also typically associated with a tonic pupil, as the ability to accommodate is typically compromised in these patients but may not be noticeable. A tonic pupil is not associated with ptosis, binocular diplopia, or severe headache and the presence of any of these symptoms should prompt further investigation into other emergent causes (e.g., third nerve palsy). Some patients however might report monocular diplopia or mild eye strain with reading (asthenopia). Although the tonic pupil is usually an isolated finding, two syndromes can also be associated with a tonic pupil, and should be considered in the differential of a patient presenting with a tonic pupil. The first syndrome is Adie syndrome (or Holmes–Adie syndrome), which consists of generalized hyporeflexia and unilateral or bilateral tonic pupils. The second syndrome is Ross syndrome, which refers to tonic pupils, hyporeflexia, and the presence of unilateral or bilateral segmental anhidrosis.[1–3] Ross syndrome can be associated with gastrointestinal (e.g., diarrhea/constipation) or cardiac (e.g., tachycardia or bradycardia) signs and thus is potentially dangerous. Although most patients with the tonic pupil are unilateral, about 4% of cases become bilateral per year and some authors consider the bilateral tonic pupil to be an indication for syphilis serology (e.g., RPR and FTA-ABS).

The solution to Question 2 is C.

The hallmarks of Adie's tonic pupil are an isolated anisocoria that is greater in the light, a dilated pupil that constricts tonically to near but does not react normally to light, sectoral or diffuse iris paresis, and denervation supersensitivity to dilute topical pilocarpine (0.1%). Ptosis (ipsilateral or contralateral) is not a sign associated with Adie's tonic pupil and in the setting of a dilated pupil its presence should prompt the clinician to the possibility of an ipsilateral third nerve palsy or a contralateral Horner syndrome, both of which may require an emergent workup (please see the chapters "Third Nerve Palsy" and "Horner Syndrome" for further discussion). Adie's tonic pupil is however commonly associated with sectoral (or segmental) iris sphincter paresis, vermiform iris movements, and/or light-near dissociation of the pupil(s). Sectoral palsy is a key feature (in addition to the absence of ptosis or motility deficit) that is useful for suggesting Adie's tonic pupil and for excluding third nerve palsy. These features, in addition to the presence of a poor pupillary reaction to light, help differentiate idiopathic Adie's tonic pupil from other causes of anisocoria. It is important to note that patients with localized iris trauma (including surgery), post-infectious (e.g., herpetic) iris or ganglion damage, or iris ischemia can also have sectoral iris palsy. The history in conjunction with slit lamp examination findings such as iris atrophy or iris transillumination defects are usually sufficient to make the diagnosis. In contrast, a pharmacologically dilated pupil would not demonstrate light-near dissociation, sectoral iris paresis, vermiform movements, or any response to dilute pilocarpine. Posterior synechiae (most commonly found in patients with a history of prior iris trauma, anterior chamber inflammation, or acute angle closure) can also mimic a tonic pupil during the initial stages but a subsequent slit lamp examination and dilated examination should help differentiate the presence or absence of synechiae and allow the clinician to distinguish between these entities.

The solution to Question 3 is B.

Topical pilocarpine testing in a patient with a fixed and dilated pupil without other signs that would indicate a third nerve palsy (i.e., motility deficits or ptosis) is especially useful for differentiating pharmacologic dilation from Adie's tonic pupil. For the diagnosis of Adie's tonic pupil, one drop of dilute pilocarpine (0.1% or 0.125% pilocarpine) OU will show constriction of the affected pupil compared to a lack of constriction in the non-affected, control pupil (assuming unilateral disease). A tonic pupil or idiopathic Adie's pupil will constrict to dilute pilocarpine due to denervation supersensitivity from an increased number of cholinergic receptors (responsible for pupillary constriction). This upregulation of the post-synaptic receptors occurs after a prolonged period of neurotransmitter deprivation following denervation. In contrast, dilute pilocarpine would typically not affect a normal pupil. Unfortunately, some normal patients (especially those with light-colored irides) may react to low-dose pilocarpine OU and thus it is important to document the results in both the affected and the control eye. It is also important, however, to note that denervation hypersensitivity has been reported in both Adie's tonic pupil as well as longstanding third nerve palsy, given their common involvement of the parasympathetic pathway.[4] Therefore, it is important to perform a complete eye examination in these patients with anisocoria as concomitant ptosis or motility deficits are the differentiating features of third nerve palsy-related mydriasis and clinicians should not rely upon the results of the dilute pilocarpine test alone for the differential diagnosis.

In contrast to topical dilute pilocarpine, the administration of 1% pilocarpine in a normal patient would be expected to demonstrate constriction of both pupils. However, a lack of response in the affected pupil would indicate a pharmacologically blocked pupil or mechanically abnormal pupil (e.g., posterior synechiae, iris atrophy, or atonic (no tone) pupil). Apraclonidine, a mixed alpha-1 and alpha-2 sympathetic agonist, is used for the diagnosis of Horner syndrome and would not be of use for parasympathetic lesions (e.g., dilated, poorly reactive pupil). Likewise, brimonidine, a primarily alpha-2 agonist, is mainly utilized for glaucoma treatment and would be expected to mildly constrict the normal pupil. In general, however, it should be emphasized that clinical examination and not topical pharmacologic testing is the key to the diagnosis in most cases of anisocoria involving the parasympathetic pathway.

The solution to Question 4 is C.

Lack of constriction of the affected pupil to both dilute and normal pilocarpine indicates the possibility of either a mechanical (e.g., iris synechiae) or pharmacologic mechanism preventing constriction of the dilated and poorly reactive pupil. A thorough history would be important to differentiate both pharmacologic and mechanical reasons of a non-reactive pupil such as recent exposure to medications associated with pupillary dilation (i.e., topical mydriatics, asthma inhalers, certain plants or flowers), or a prior history of ocular trauma or surgery. A thorough slit lamp examination would be equally important in evaluating between these causes. No other slit lamp exam abnormalities would be expected with pharmacologic dilation. In contrast, if there is evidence of anterior inflammation (posterior synechiae, anterior chamber cell or flare), iris damage (e.g., sphincter tear), iris transillumination defects (iris atrophy), or iris ischemia (e.g., markedly elevated intraocular pressure in acute angle closure), then pharmacologic dilation would be less likely although multiple mechanisms are sometimes present (e.g., a patient is on topical mydriatics after post-surgical cases or after treatment for uveitis). Posterior synechiae can occur despite mydriatics and produce anisocoria following a red eye (e.g., uveitis). A pupil with this mechanical mydriasis would not constrict to topical pilocarpine of any strength and would not react to light or near stimuli or show a consensual response. Fortunately, the slit lamp examination is typically diagnostic for posterior synechiae, obviating the need for imaging.

Light-near dissociation could be associated with a variety of mechanisms including Adie's tonic pupil, longstanding third nerve palsy with aberrant regeneration, non-Adie-related tonic pupils, or even wearing off of pharmacologic dilation. Segmental iris sphincter paresis is most consistent with Adie's tonic pupil but should respond to both dilute (if denervation supersensitivity is present) and normal-strength pilocarpine in both eyes. Therefore, the dilute pilocarpine should be given before the normal-strength pilocarpine in Adie's tonic pupil. The constriction of the affected pupil to the consensual light reflex would be unlikely in cases of efferent (iris) pupil abnormalities but light-near dissociation of the pupils can occur (without anisocoria) in afferent pupillary disease. For example, a pupil in a patient with poor vision (no light perception) might not respond to light but will demonstrate a normal reaction to near (efferent testing); but even a patient with no light perception vision in one eye will not have anisocoria due to the intact consensual pupillary response. In the patient presented at the beginning of this case, the lack of pupillary response to 1% pilocarpine localizes the pupillary dysfunction to the efferent pathway (located at the iris in this example). Ptosis and motility deficits are the hallmark of third nerve palsy and these findings do not occur in Adie's tonic pupil or pharmacologic dilation.

The solution to Question 5 is A.

To determine which pupil is abnormal in a case of anisocoria, the pupils should be measured in both the light and dark. If the anisocoria is greater in the light, the eye with the larger dilated pupil is most likely to be the affected eye. Although multiple etiologies can cause a dilated pupil, the presence of a severe headache as an associated symptom should prompt a workup to rule out potentially dangerous or life-threatening causes, such as an enlarging intracranial aneurysm presenting with an acute third nerve palsy. Thus, it is important that in any patient presenting with anisocoria with a dilated pupil, extra care is taken to examine both the lids for ptosis and extraocular motility for any deficits that may be suggestive of a cranial nerve palsy.[5] Visual acuity and visual field measurements, the presence or absence of an RAPD, and the dilated fundus examination are all essential components of a complete eye examination but unfortunately would not differentiate between various efferent causes of a dilated pupil. Exophthalmometer measurements, while helpful in suspected orbital or thyroid eye disease, would not help differentiate the etiology of a dilated pupil. Light-near dissociation unfortunately can occur in third nerve palsy cases with aberrant regeneration. Topical pilocarpine likewise is useful for differentiating pharmacologic dilation (no response to pilocarpine) from third nerve palsy (response to pilocarpine) when used to compare between the affected eye with the fellow, normal pupil as a control.

The solution to Question 6 is B.

The patient's history of recent surgery is particularly important, given that her large pupil is acute, isolated, and non-reactive to light, which is highly suggestive of a pharmacologic etiology. However, to evaluate for any potentially dangerous etiologies that can also be associated with large pupil anisocoria, the remainder of the clinical exam is very important. Even if pharmacologic dilation is suspected, it is still important to evaluate both the lids and extraocular motility of the affected eye in all diagnostic positions of gaze to identify any cranial nerve III involvement.

In a patient presenting with pupillary block, the pupil is typically mid-dilated with other signs and symptoms of angle closure glaucoma, such as a markedly hyperemic eye, increased intraocular pressure, and evidence on slit lamp exam demonstrating iris sphincter approximation to the anterior lens capsule with or without posterior synechiae. Although benign episodic mydriasis can cause a dilated pupil, it is often associated with young, otherwise healthy females and migraine headaches, comes and goes intermittently, and presents with only mild symptoms of blurring or is asymptomatic and noticed by the patient or family member.[5,6] In addition, in benign episodic mydriasis, the pupil would not typically remain completely non-reactive and usually is not as widely dilated as is seen with pharmacologic dilation.

An effective test to help differentiate the various etiologies of a dilated pupil in this patient would include the use of topical pilocarpine (diluted 0.1 or 0.125% first, and then 1% if no response to the diluted concentration) applied to both eyes (using the non-affected eye as a control). Constriction of both the affected and non-affected pupils would be expected in a patient with a third nerve palsy or benign episodic mydriasis, but not in a patient with pharmacologic dilation.[7] In the setting of pharmacologic mydriasis, it is also important to obtain a clear and careful history to identify the cause of the mydriasis, which can be due to rubbing of the eye following contact with an anticholinergic substance (e.g., scopolamine patch is most common post-surgery).[6]

SUMMARY

A large pupil with anisocoria should be evaluated in a clear, systematic, and methodical manner. It is important in any patient with large pupil anisocoria to evaluate for other abnormalities in the ocular examination, especially the lid and extraocular motility, to rule out the possibility of a third nerve palsy. Closer examination at the slit lamp can help differentiate the different etiologies of a dilated pupil, including segmental iris sphincter paresis, vermiform iris movements, light-near dissociation, iris atrophy, anterior chamber inflammation, posterior synechiae, or obvious iris trauma. Large pupil anisocoria can be caused by multiple etiologies including a tonic pupil (Adie's tonic pupil), posterior synechiae, iris trauma or ischemia, a pharmacologically dilated pupil, third nerve palsy, or benign episodic unilateral mydriasis. To help differentiate these different etiologies, the use of dilute (0.1% or 0.125%) and normal-strength pilocarpine (1%) may be helpful, as long as the contralateral eye is used as a control and the testing is interpreted accurately in coordination with the other clinical exam findings. Tonic pupils can also be associated with certain systemic syndromes including Holmes–Adie (or Adie) syndrome (generalized hyporeflexia) and Ross syndrome (associated with tonic pupils, generalized hyporeflexia, and segmental anhidrosis) or rarely syphilis.

REFERENCES

1. Kelly-Sell M, Liu GT. (2011) "Tonic" but not "Adie" pupils. *J Neuroophthalmol* **31**:393–395.
2. Yasar S, Aslan C, Serdar ZA, *et al.* (2010) Ross syndrome: unilateral hyperhidrosis, Adie's tonic pupils and diffuse areflexia. *J Dtsch Dermatol Ges* **8**:1004–1006.
3. Bremner FD, Smith SE. (2007) Bilateral tonic pupils: Holmes-Adie syndrome or generalised neuropathy? *Br J Ophthalmol* **91**:1620–1623.
4. Jacobson DM, Vierkant RA. (1998) Comparison of cholinergic supersensitivity in third nerve palsy and Adie's syndrome. *J Neuroophthalmol* **18**:171–175.
5. Lee AG, Taber KH, Hayman LA, Tang RA. (1997) A guide to the isolated dilated pupil. *Arch Fam Med* **6**:385–388.
6. Moeller JJ, Maxner CE. (2007) The dilated pupil: an update. *Curr Neurol Neurosci Rep* **7**:417–422.
7. Wilhelm H. (1998) Neuro-ophthalmology of pupillary function — practical guidelines. *J Neurol* **245**:573–583.

3

Toxic/Nutritional Optic Neuropathy

Nagham Al-Zubidi MD, Rick N. Nordgren MD, Arielle Spitze MD, Sushma Yalamanchili MD, and Andrew G. Lee MD

CASE

A 30-year-old Indian man reported difficulty using a camera with his left eye for several years. He denied any toxic exposure (e.g., poisons, heavy metals, or chemicals). He was not a vegan and reported eating three meals per day. He denied any vomiting, anorexia, or bariatric surgery. There was no history of tuberculosis (TB) or treatment with anti-TB medications (e.g., isoniazid or ethambutol). He denied any other neurological symptoms except for mild photophobia. The remainder of his medical, surgical, and social history was unremarkable. On examination, his best-corrected visual acuity was 20/20–2 in the right eye (OD) and 20/60–2 in the left eye (OS). Pupils were 4 mm in the dark and 2 mm in the light and there was a left relative afferent pupillary defect (RAPD). He correctly identified 8/8 Ishihara color plates OD but only 1.5/8 OS. The extraocular movements, intraocular pressures, and slit lamp examinations were normal bilaterally (OU). Dilated funduscopic examination demonstrated mild temporal pallor OU (Fig. 3.1). Automated visual fields (Humphrey 24-2) demonstrated a mild bilateral central scotomas OS > OD (Fig. 3.2). Magnetic resonance imaging (MRI) of the brain and orbits with and without gadolinium and fat suppression were normal and demonstrated no optic nerve enhancement or compressive lesion. Optical coherence tomography (OCT) showed papillomacular bundle nerve fiber layer dropout OU.

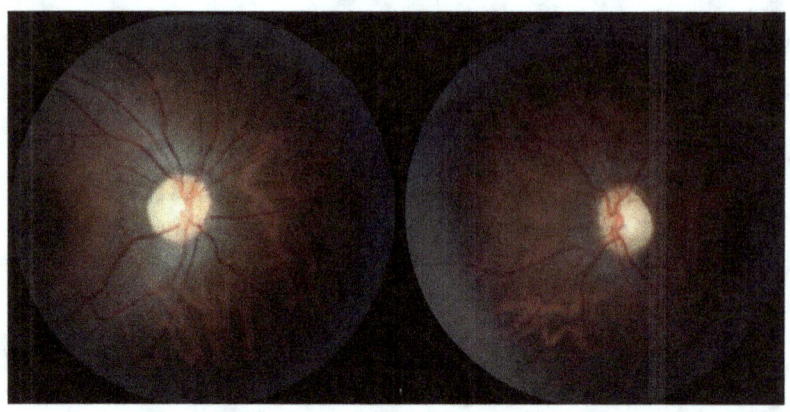

Fig. 3.1. Fundus photographs demonstrating a mild temporal pallor OU.

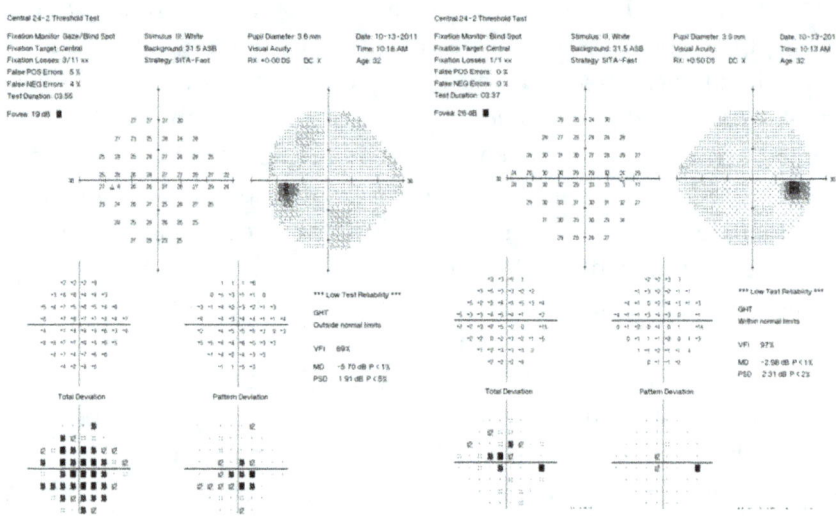

Fig. 3.2. Automated visual fields (Humphrey 24-2) demonstrating a mild bilateral central scotoma OS > OD.

Question 1	Question 2
Which of the following symptoms is most consistent with typical nutritional optic neuropathy?	**Which of the following signs is most consistent with nutritional optic neuropathy?**
A. Acute bilateral painful central vision loss B. Progressive unilateral painful vision loss C. Acute painless peripheral vision loss D. Progressive bilateral central vision loss	A. RAPD with temporal pallor OD only B. Bilateral cecocentral scotomas C. Disc pallor OD and disc edema OS D. Bilateral optic disc edema
Question 3	Question 4
Which of the following vitamin deficiencies is the most likely cause of nutritional optic neuropathy in the US?	**Which of the following drugs is most likely to produce a toxic optic neuropathy?**
A. Vitamin B1 (thiamine) B. Vitamin B2 (riboflavin) C. Vitamin B6 (pyridoxine) D. Vitamin B12 (cyanocobalamin)	A. Hydroxychloroquine B. Tamoxifen C. Ethambutol D. Penicillamine
Question 5	Question 6
Which of the following types of bilateral visual field defects is most likely in toxic/nutritional optic neuropathy?	**Which of the following nerve fibers are most affected in toxic/nutritional optic neuropathy?**
A. Altitudinal field defect B. Bitemporal hemianopsia C. Cecocentral scotomas D. Homonymous hemianopsia	A. Papillomacular fibers B. Superior temporal fibers C. Inferior temporal fibers D. Superior and inferior nasal fibers

Question 7	Question 8
Which of the following is the next most appropriate step in a patient with nutritional optic neuropathy and a borderline low normal B12 level and low folate level?	Which of the following antibody tests is most likely to be positive in a patient with B12 deficiency-related optic neuropathy?
A. Give folate replacement only B. MRI of the head and orbit with contrast C. Leber hereditary optic neuropathy test D. Serum methylmalonic acid	A. Tissue transglutaminase B. Intrinsic factor antibodies C. Endomysial antibody test D. Gliadin antibodies
Question 9	Question 10
Which of the following conditions is most likely in a young man with acute bilateral cecocentral scotomas and then temporal pallor OU?	Which of the following substance abuse problems is most likely in a patient with nutritional optic neuropathy?
A. Leber hereditary optic neuropathy B. Rod /cone dystrophy C. Compressive optic neuropathy D. Retrochiasmal lesions	A. Ethanol B. Cocaine C. Heroin D. Toluene

EXPLANATIONS

The solution to Question 1 is D.

Most toxic/nutritional optic neuropathies develop slowly over time (months) with a painless, bilateral, symmetric, progressive loss of central vision (i.e., loss of visual acuity and central/cecocentral scotomas) often accompanied by color vision deficits. The vision loss is typically bilateral, central, and symmetric due to the systemic nature of the problem (toxin or nutritional deficiency); however, in some cases the presentation may be asymmetric especially early in the course.[1] Some cases of toxic optic neuropathy may present with acute, bilateral, and severe vision loss such as poisoning with methanol or ethylene glycol. Pain, strictly unilateral findings, an acute onset, the presence of atypical visual field defects (not typical central/cecocentral scotomas), or the presence of optic disc edema should prompt consideration for alternative etiologies other than toxic/-nutritional optic neuropathy. Leber hereditary optic neuropathy (LHON) can present acutely with a bilateral simultaneous or sequential central or cecocentral visual loss and should be in the differential diagnosis in patients with suspected toxic/nutritional optic neuropathy, especially in those patients who do not respond to treatment and/or discontinuation of the offending toxin.

The solution to Question 2 is B.

Nutritional and toxic optic neuropathies predominantly affect the papillomacular bundle but it remains unclear why these particular fibers are selectively affected. The papillomacular bundle from the macula exits the eye at the temporal aspect of the optic disc, and damage to these fibers will cause a central or cecocentral scotoma and eventual temporal pallor of the optic discs. Since the color-sensitive cones are at their highest concentration in the macula patients often present with early and ultimately more severe color vision deficits. In fact, subtle color vision changes may be the first clinical sign of optic neuropathy in these patients.[1] As noted above in Question 1, toxic/nutritional optic neuropathies most commonly present in a bilateral and symmetric fashion, therefore typically no RAPD will be appreciated; however, the pupillary response may be sluggish bilaterally. An RAPD may be present however in bilateral but asymmetric disease. Optic disc edema is uncommon in nutritional optic neuropathy and is usually only seen in combination with acute toxin exposure.[2] Unilateral optic disc edema with contralateral optic atrophy can be due to the Foster Kennedy syndrome with a compressive mass lesion on one side and papilledema from increased intracranial pressure in the fellow eye. The pseudo–Foster Kennedy syndrome results from unilateral, acute optic disc edema from non-arteritic anterior ischemic optic neuropathy (NAION) in one eye and optic atrophy from prior NAION in the fellow eye.

The solution to Question 3 is D.

Vitamin B_{12} has an important role in the maintenance of the nervous system function. In the developed world, a poor diet (e.g., alcohol abuse, strict vegan, eating disorder) can cause vitamin B_{12} deficiency, but patients who have undergone bariatric or other gastrointestinal surgery may also be at risk. Pernicious anemia is an autoimmune disorder producing impaired intrinsic factor function and impaired vitamin B_{12} absorption.[3]

Although multiple vitamin deficiencies often occur together due to a common etiology (e.g., alcohol abuse, poor nutrition, gastric surgery), folate and B_{12} deficiency are the most common causes for nutritional optic neuropathy in the United States. Thiamine deficiency produces the Wernicke syndrome and can present acutely with ophthalmoplegia or nystagmus.

The solution to Question 4 is C.

Ethambutol produces a dose-dependent toxic optic neuropathy. Ethambutol is used in the treatment of tuberculosis (and other atypical mycobacteria) and is a bacteriostatic antimicrobial agent. The exact mechanism of action is unclear; however, it is thought to be a chelating agent that binds to and disrupts enzymes located in the nucleic acid structure of the bacteria. The incidence of toxic optic neuropathy from ethambutol toxicity ranges from 1–5% depending on dose and duration. In contrast to most toxic optic neuropathies, the visual symptoms can begin early and often start within two to eight months after initiation of the drug. Some authors believe that the earliest sign of visual dysfunction is dyschromatopsia (especially blue–yellow).[4,5] The most common visual field defects, as in other toxic/nutritional optic neuropathies, are bilateral central or cecocentral scotomas but peripheral forms exist as well. Nerve fiber layer thinning can be seen using OCT analysis of the optic disc and may appear prior to obvious changes in the appearance of the fundus. Although ethambutol is thought to produce visual loss through an optic neuropathy other testing (e.g., multifocal electroretinogram) has shown evidence for concomitant retinal toxicity as well.[6] When ethambutol toxicity is suspected the drug should be discontinued and some patients may still recover normal visual function. One Korean study however demonstrated that only a minority of patients recovered visual function despite stopping the drug and that visual recovery is less likely to occur if significant optic disc pallor is already present. Thus, early recognition and discontinuation of the medication are critical before the development of irreversible optic atrophy. The toxicity of ethambutol is dose dependent and many patients receive up to 25 mg/kg daily for the first two months and then are recommended to decrease to a dose of 15 mg/kg thereafter. Unfortunately, toxicity can still occur at these lower dosage levels and vigilance is required.[6] Patients starting ethambutol should receive an initial screening ophthalmic evaluation including visual field, color vision, dilated funduscopic exam, and visual acuity and other baseline screening modalities may include OCT of the optic nerve to document and detect early nerve fiber layer loss. Monthly examinations are recommended for patients on ethambutol who are at a higher risk of toxicity.[7,8] The additional risk factors for toxicity include diabetes mellitus, chronic renal failure, alcoholism, old age, young age (children), other ocular defects, ethambutol-induced peripheral neuropathy, and a dose greater than 15 mg/kg/day.[9]

Although lower plasma zinc levels have been associated with a higher risk of developing toxicity, excessive zinc can interfere with the metabolism of copper and cause other side effects. Therefore, although patients with a low serum zinc level might benefit from supplementation treatment there is no clear evidence-based recommendation that can be made at this time for zinc in ethambutol toxicity.[10] Hydroxychloroquine can cause central and paracentral visual loss due to a bull's eye maculopathy OU. Tamoxifen produces a crystalline retinopathy. Penicillamine can produce myasthenia gravis.

The solution to Question 5 is C.

Although the mechanism of toxicity is not known, the nerve fibers supplying the papillomacular bundle are often selectively affected in toxic/nutritional optic neuropathy. Damage to these fibers leads to central or cecocentral visual field defects as seen in our patient in this case. Other visual field defects are possible such as peripheral defects (e.g., peripheral toxicity) or even pseudo-bitemporal hemianopsia in ethambutol toxicity from breakout of the central or cecocentral scotoma into the temporal periphery OU.[11]

In contrast to a pure bitemporal hemianopsia, patients with the pseudo-bitemporal hemianopsia of ethambutol toxicity have loss of central visual field and visual acuity. Chiasmal toxicity however has been postulated in some toxic visual loss. Altitudinal visual field loss is more typical of optic neuropathies that spare rather than involve the papillomacular bundle (e.g., glaucoma, chronic papilledema, disc drusen). A homonymous hemianopsia localizes to the contralateral retrochiasmal pathway and would not be expected in toxic/nutritional optic neuropathy.

The solution to Question 6 is A (see above).

The solution to Question 7 is D.

A borderline or low serum B_{12} level may still signify a symptomatic and pathologic B_{12} deficiency that can be a treatable cause of nutritional optic neuropathy. In order to confirm a more longstanding B_{12} deficiency in this setting, plasma homocysteine and methylmalonic acid levels should also be considered. This is particularly important for borderline B_{12} levels as both homocysteine and methylmalonic acid will be elevated from longer-term deficiency states. If only homocysteine is elevated then a concomitant folate deficiency may be present instead. Cobalamin (B_{12}) is involved in the conversion of homocysteine to methionine as well as the conversion of methylmalonyl-CoA to succinyl-CoA. Folate is involved in the methylation of cobalamin (to methylcobalamin) that in turn methylates homocysteine to create methionine. Folate however is not involved in the conversion of methylmalonyl-CoA to succinyl-CoA.[12] Red blood cell (RBC) folate is also recommended by some authors as the serum folate may be artifactually normal even in deficiency states.[13] Supplementation with B_{12} and folate as well as a search for the underlying etiology for the deficiency state is important and ophthalmologists should probably refer these patients back to the primary care physician for evaluation and treatment as well as follow-up vitamin levels. Patients with a bilateral, progressive optic neuropathy who do not have B_{12} or folate deficiency documented as the cause might still require further testing including MRI, lumbar puncture, or LHON testing. In general however patients with a typical toxic/nutritional etiology do not require these additional tests if there is a defined etiology and the patient responds to treatment.

The solution to Question 8 is B.

Vitamin B_{12} is absorbed in the ileum after being bound to intrinsic factor in the duodenum. Intrinsic factor is secreted by the gastric parietal cells. Therefore, auto-antibodies to either intrinsic factor or parietal cells can lead to poor vitamin B_{12} absorption and subsequent B_{12} deficiency.[14] Auto-antibodies are found in autoimmune gastritis and pernicious anemia. Pernicious anemia is also associated with other autoimmune disease important for the ophthalmic history, namely autoimmune thyroid disease and type I diabetes mellitus.[15]

Ophthalmologists who diagnose toxic/nutritional optic neuropathy should recommend discontinuation of smoking/alcohol use and refer the patient back to the primary care physician for evaluation and treatment of any underlying etiology including nutritional deficiency or pernicious anemia. Anti-tissue transglutaminase (tTG-IgA), anti-endomysial (EMA-IgA), and anti-gliadin antibodies (AGA-IgG and AGA-IgA) may be seen in celiac disease and other inflammatory bowel disorders but would not generally be ordered by the ophthalmologist.

The solution to Question 9 is A.

Leber hereditary optic neuropathy is associated with specific genetic mutations to human mitochondrial DNA (e.g., positions 11778, 3460, and 14484).[16,17] These mutations lead to dysfunctional adenosine triphosphate (ATP) production due to defects in oxidative phosphorylation especially in highly energy-dependent tissues such as the optic nerve. The most common mutation in LHON is at the

11778 location. Patients with the 14484 mutation have the highest chance for visual improvement after the initial loss of vision.[18]

There is evidence suggesting that vision loss in LHON may be precipitated by environmental factors including nutritional deprivation, smoking, alcohol consumption, psychological stress, and acute illness. The typical patient with LHON is a young male with acute, bilateral, simultaneous or rapidly sequential central/cecocentral scotomas. The optic nerve may appear swollen initially (pseudoedema) or have peripapillary telangiectasias (LHON fundus) and then over time the optic nerve develops temporal pallor OU. Although there is no proven treatment for LHON, vitamin supplementation and treatment with Coenzyme Q10 (Co-Q_{10}) and its derivatives has been advocated by some. As LHON is a maternally inherited mitochondrial disorder the affected male cannot transmit LHON but maternal-side relatives are at risk of harboring or transmitting the disease.

Rod-cone or cone dystrophies would not be expected to present acutely but could mimic the presentation of LHON with a chronic bilateral central/cecocentral scotoma and an initially normal fundus exam in a young patient. Multifocal electroretinogram (MERG) might confirm central retinal dysfunction. Compressive lesions can mimic a bilateral retrobulbar optic neuropathy and rarely might present with a central/cecocentral scotoma, and a normal fundus exam and an imaging study should be considered in patients with suspected LHON or toxic/nutritional optic neuropathy for whom the diagnosis is not secure. A unilateral retrochiasmal lesion would not produce central/cecocentral scotomas OU; a bilateral retrochiasmal lesion (e.g., bilateral occipital tip infarction) however might mimic a central scotoma which actually is a bilateral but juxtaposed macular-involving homonymous paracentral hemianopsia.

The solution to Question 10 is A.

Excessive alcohol use is a major cause of nutritional deficiency by both its effects on the intake and metabolism of nutrients and end organ damage. A rapid fall in serum folate can occur within two to four days of alcohol abuse by impairing its enterohepatic cycle and inhibiting its absorption. This period is shorter than normal in part because alcoholics start with lower stores due to previous dietary habits.[12] Some authors have advocated for measuring red blood cell folate over serum folate alone because eating a single folate-rich meal can artifactually raise the acutely measured serum folate level (versus RBC folate which reflects chronic deficiency). The RBC folate assay however may have less specificity and sensitivity and RBC folate levels may be decreased in up to 63% of patients with vitamin B_{12} deficiency.[19] In one study, three tests were evaluated from 45 laboratories: (1) serum folate only (42%), (2) RBC folate only (45%), and (3) both assays (12.5%). Of 1355 samples, 57 had low RBC folate results but in only 3 of these 57 samples (5%) were there a change in clinical outcome (i.e., serum folate was normal, RBC folate was low, and the patient responded to folate supplementation therapy). The authors concluded that the RBC folate assay provided no additional clinical information for > 95% of patients and that serum folate assay was the most appropriate screening test to detect folic acid deficiency.[13] As noted with borderline B_{12} deficiency, an elevation of plasma methylmalonic acid and homocysteine may be a more sensitive and better indicator of functional deficiency producing a toxic/nutritional optic neuropathy than relying upon folate levels alone. Our patient was found to be B_{12}-deficient with normal folate level, IF and parietal cell antibodies were positive and a diagnosis of pernicious anemia was made. He was treated with supplementation therapy and his visual function stabilized.

SUMMARY

Toxic/nutritional optic neuropathy causes painless, progressive, bilateral, central, and symmetric vision loss, predominantly affects the optic nerve fibers to the papillomacular bundle, and causes a central or cecocentral scotoma and temporal pallor. Nutritional optic neuropathies are often associated with deficiencies in specific vitamins (e.g., vitamin B_{12} and RBC folate). Ethambutol is a common cause of toxic optic neuropathy and early recognition and discontinuation of the drug is critical to prevent irreversible blindness.

REFERENCES

1. Orssaud C, Roche O, Dufier JL. (2007) Nutritional optic neuropathies. *J Neurol Sci* **262**:158–164.

2. Sharma P, Sharma R. (2011) Toxic optic neuropathy. *Indian J Ophthalmol* **59**:137–141.

3. Phillips PH. (2005) Toxic and deficiency optic neuropathies. In: Miller NR, Newman NJ, Biousse V, Kerrison JB (eds), *Walsh and Hoyt's Clinical Neuro-Ophthalmology*. Lippincott Williams & Wilkins, Philadelphia, PA, pp. 447–453.

4. Polak BC, Leys M, van Lith GH. (1985) Blue-yellow colour vision changes as early symptoms of ethambutol oculotoxicity. *Ophthalmologica* **191**:223–226.

5. Chai SJ, Foroozan R. (2007) Decreased retinal nerve fiber layer thickness detected by optical coherence tomography in patients with ethambutol-induced optic neuropathy. *Br J Ophthalmol* **91**:895–897.

6. Mathur KC, Sankhla JS. (1976) Ophthalmic manifestations of the toxicity of ethambutol. *Indian J Ophthalmol* **24**:6–9.

7. Lee EJ, Kim SJ, Choung HK, *et al.* (2008) Incidence and clinical features of ethambutol-induced optic neuropathy in Korea. *J Neuroophthalmol* **28**: 269–277.

8. Griffith DE, Brown-Elliott BA, Shepherd S, *et al.* (2005) Ethambutol ocular toxicity in treatment regimens for Mycobacterium avium complex lung disease. *Am J Respir Crit Care Med* **172**:250–253.

9. Fraunfelder FW, Fraunfelder FT. (2012) Drug-related adverse effects of clinical importance to the ophthalmologist. AAO course 313, November.

10. Miller NR, Newman NJ, Biousse V, Kerrison JB, eds. (2005) *Walsh and Hoyt's Clinical Neuro-Ophthalmology*, 6th ed. Lippincott Williams & Wilkins, Philadelphia, PA.

11. Lim SA. (2006) Ethambutol-associated optic neuropathy. *Ann Acad Med Singapore* **35**:274–278.

12. Antony AC. (2005) Megaloblastic anemias. In: Hoffman R, Benz EJ Jr, Shattil SJ, *et al.* (eds), *Hematology: Basic Principles and Practice*, 4th ed. Churchill Livingston, New York, NY, p. 519.

13. Galloway M, Rushworth L. (2003) Red cell or serum folate? Results from the National Pathology Alliance benchmarking review. *J Clin Pathol* **56**:924–926.

14. Toh BH, van Driel IR, Gleeson PA. (1997) Pernicious anemia. *N Engl J Med* **337**: 1441–1448.

15. Stabler SP. (2013) Clinical practice. Vitamin B12 deficiency. *N Engl J Med* **368**: 149–160.

16. Man PYM, Turnbull DM, Chinnery PF. (2002) Leber hereditary optic neuropathy. *J Med Genet* **39**:162–169.

17. Jun AS, Brown MD, Wallace DC. (1994) A mitochondrial DNA mutation at nucleotide pair 14459 of the NADH dehydrogenase subunit 6 gene associated with maternally inherited Leber hereditary optic neuropathy and dystonia. *Proc Natl Acad Sci USA* **91**: 6206–6210.
18. Riordan-Eva P, Sanders MD, Govan GG, *et al.* (1995) The clinical features of Leber's hereditary optic neuropathy defined by the presence of a pathogenic mitochondrial DNA mutation. *Brain* **118**: 319–337.

4

Optic Disc Drusen

Nagham Al-Zubidi MD, James D. Kim MD,
Arielle Spitze MD, and Andrew G. Lee MD

CASE

A 35-year-old female presented with transient visual obscurations (TVOs) in the left eye (OS) that lasted 5–15 seconds at a time. Her symptoms began three months ago and occurred approximately every three weeks. They were triggered by stress and fatigue, but resolved with rest. She denied any headaches or diplopia. The rest of her past medical, surgical, social, and family histories were non-contributory. There was no prior history of migraine. On examination the best-corrected visual acuity was 20/25 in both eyes (OU). Pupils measured 5 mm in the dark OU, 3 mm in the light OU, with a relative afferent pupillary defect measuring 0.3 log units OS. Color vision test with Ishihara color plates was 14 out of 14 plates OU. Extraocular motility was full. Intraocular pressure measurements and slit lamp examination were within normal limits. Dilated funduscopic examination was normal except for the optic discs OU as shown in Fig. 4.1. The automated perimetry (Humphrey 24-2) is shown in Fig. 4.2.

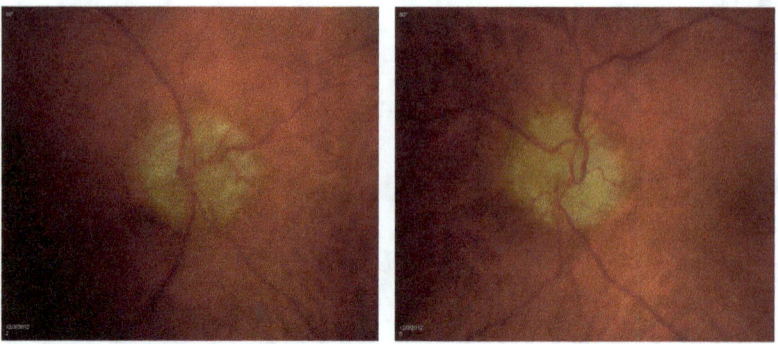

Fig. 4.1. Optic disc photographs of the patient. Note the blurred margin and lumpy-bumpy refractile bodies within the disc head.

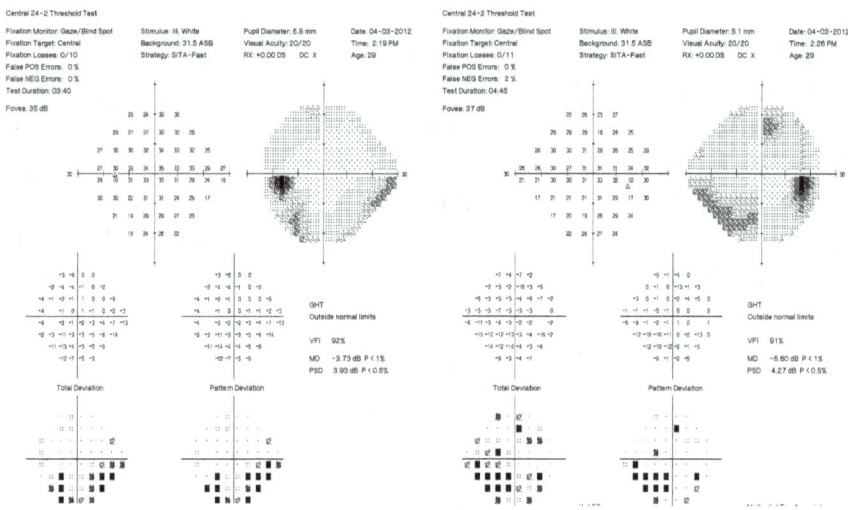

Fig. 4.2. Automated perimetry of the patient. Note the inferonasal visual field defect bilaterally.

Question 1	Question 2
Which of the following findings is most likely to be present in a patient with optic nerve head drusen?	Which of the following findings is most consistent with optic disc drusen (ODD)?
A. Acute vision loss B. Central scotoma C. Asymptomatic D. Optic disc edema	A. Loss of central visual acuity B. Transient visual obscurations C. Obscuration of nerve fiber layer D. Pulsatile tinnitus
Question 3	Question 4
Which of the following is the most sensitive and specific initial imaging modality for detection of calcified ODD?	Which of the following best represents the percentage of patients with ODD with visual field loss?
A. Magnetic resonance imaging of orbit B. Fluorescein angiography C. Ultrasound of the optic nerve D. Optical coherence tomography	A. 95% B. 75% C. 25% D. 15%
Question 5	Question 6
Which of the following findings is most likely in a patient with ODD?	Which of the following ultrasonographic findings is more likely to be found in true papilledema compared to ODD?
A. Hemianopic visual field loss B. Nerve fiber layer defects C. Macular exudates D. Decreased visual acuity	A. Elevation of the optic nerve head B. Negative 30-degree test C. Increased fluid in the optic sheath D. High reflectivity signal in the optic nerve with gain turned down low

Question 7	Question 8
Which of the following is the most likely visual field loss pattern in a patient with ODD?	**Which of the following signs is a feature of true disc edema but not ODD?**
A. Arcuate visual field defect **B.** Cecocentral scotoma **C.** Central scotoma **D.** Bitemporal hemianopsia	**A.** Elevated optic discs **B.** Obscured peripapillary nerve fiber layer **C.** Hyperfluorescent staining on fundus fluorescein angiography (FFA). **D.** Negative 30-degree test
Question 9	
Which of the following is the best management of a patient with visual field loss due to ODD?	
A. Coenzyme Q_{10} **B.** Serial visual fields **C.** Optic nerve sheath fenestration **D.** Glaucoma surgery	

EXPLANATIONS

The solution to Question 1 is C. The solution to Question 2 is B.

Optic disc drusen are acellular, benign, often calcified deposits in the optic disc which are presumed to be caused by axoplasmic transport alteration and axonal degeneration. The ODD result in a crowded appearance of the optic discs and they may be associated with congenital anomalous optic disc head vasculature with increased branching and increased number of vessels. ODD occur in up to 3.4–24 cases per 1,000 in the general population. They are bilateral in 75% of the cases. The number and size of ODD are highly variable and ODD are often buried within the disc. This can present as pseudopapilledema especially in children as the ODD tend to be buried in younger patients. Most patients with ODD are asymptomatic but some may present after an insidious and slowly progressive nerve fiber-type peripheral visual field loss. Acute presentations including loss of central acuity or central visual field loss due to ischemic complications are rare but reported. ODD can mimic true papilledema and the diagnosis of pseudo-papilledema in the setting of ODD is important in order to avoid unnecessary workup. Ultrasound might be diagnostic for calcified drusen but atypical features should prompt neuroimaging (e.g., rapidly progressive or acute visual field defects or central visual loss).[1-3] Transient visual obscurations lasting seconds at a time (similar to those seen in papilledema) may occur in patients with ODD. Other symptoms such as pulse-synchronous tinnitus, headache, diplopia from non-localizing sixth nerve palsy, or other signs of increased intracranial pressure, however, should not be present. An elevated optic disc with a blurred disc margin is seen in true papilledema as well as pseudo-papilledema from ODD and it is not a differentiating sign. In our opinion, the vague and non-differentiating description of "blurred disc margin" should probably be replaced with the more specific ophthalmoscopic description of the peripapillary nerve fiber layer with or without obscuration (a sign of true disc edema) and the presence of any obligatory signs of pathology (e.g., hemorrhage, exudates, cotton wool patch, retinal nerve fiber layer edema, or subretinal fluid).

The solution to Question 3 is C.

ODD appear as hyperechoic signals within the optic nerve on B-scan orbital echography (Fig. 4.3).[4] This hyperechoic signal can persist even with the ultrasound gain turned down. Unfortunately, even though ultrasonography is the most sensitive of the diagnostic tests for evaluation of buried calcified drusen, the overall sensitivity of the test for ODD is only approximately 50% because of non-calcified ODD. Computed tomography (CT) can also detect calcified ODD as a hyperdensity due to calcium content, but CT is more expensive and it is not as sensitive for ODD as the B-scan ultrasound. In addition, routine CT scan has a slice thickness of 1.5 mm and it might potentially miss smaller or non-calcified ODD.[5] Furthermore, higher costs and exposure to radiation (especially in children) make CT less suitable for routine detection of ODD. ODD can be autofluorescent (on

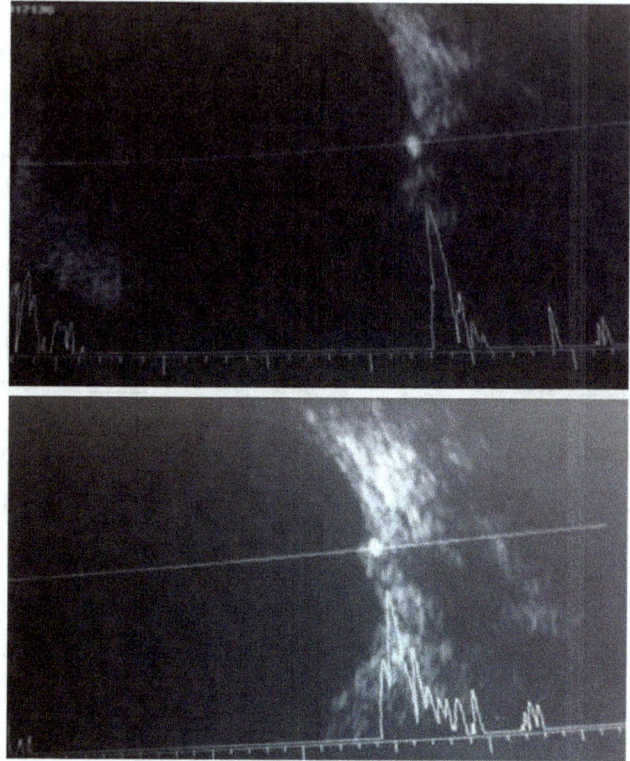

Fig. 4.3. Humphrey visual field showing optic disc drusen as a hyperechoic structure within the optic nerve.

pre-injection fluorescein angiography) and buried ODD can sometimes be detected by fluorescein angiography (FA) as staining without leakage compared with the hyperfluorescent leakage of true optic disc edema (Fig. 4.4). However, the sensitivity of pre-injection FA for ODD is still lower than that of B-scan and most cases of hyperfluorescent ODD can be seen ophthalmoscopically.[5] Optical coherence tomography (OCT) can be used to measure the retinal nerve fiber layer (RNFL) thinning seen in ODD versus RNFL thickening seen in true optic disc edema. Recent studies of spectral domain OCT have also shown unique features of ODD including the homogeneous nature of the calcified internal component of optic disc drusen but

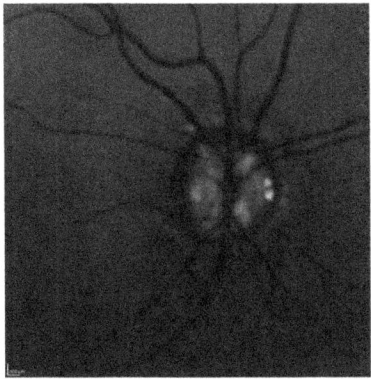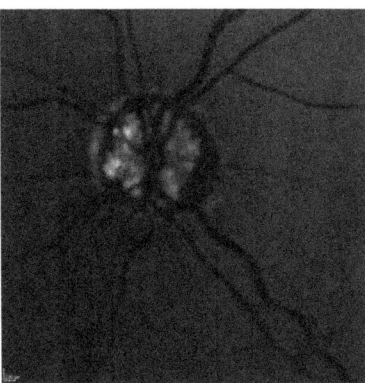

Fig. 4.4. Pre-injection fluorescein angiogram showing autofluorescence of the optic disc drusen.

have not been sufficiently validated in our opinion yet to replace ultrasonography as the procedure of choice for ODD.[6]

The solution to Question 4 is B.

Visual field defects on automated perimetry are found in approximately 75% of patients with ODD including asymptomatic patients. Mustonen examined 307 eyes with verified superficial and buried ODD and found that 224 eyes (73.4%) demonstrated visual field defect.[7] However, the true incidence of visual field defects in ODD is difficult to accurately measure because asymptomatic patients may not seek medical attention.

The solution to Question 5 is B.

The refractile bodies of the superficial and buried ODD often increase in size and become more visible over the years but this finding may not be associated with a further deterioration of the visual field.[8] The visual field defects of ODD include enlargement of the blind spot, arcuate defects, inferonasal and inferotemporal defects. There are several hypotheses to explain the origin of ODD and series of histochemical studies have shown that ODD may originate from axoplasmic flow stasis and metabolic derivatives of slowly degenerating nerve fibers.[3] Chronic true optic disc edema may cause accumulation of exudates that can superficially resemble ODD (i.e., pseudodrusen). However, these pseudodrusen are smaller, more refractile, and usually disappear over time after resolution of optic disc edema. ODD does not affect central visual acuity in the majority of patients unless it is end-stage (similar to glaucoma), accompanied by an ischemic event (e.g., non-arteritic anterior ischemic optic neuropathy), or an additional unrelated cause for the visual loss (e.g., maculopathy, optic neuropathy). In a study by Mustonen, only 2 out of 307 eyes had impaired visual acuity due to ODD.[7,8] We recommend neuroimaging for patients with ODD who have unexplained central visual field or acuity loss or any atypical, non-nerve fiber layer (e.g., hemianopic) visual field loss.

The solution to Question 6 is C.

The A-scan ultrasound can be utilized to precisely measure the quantitative thickness of the optic nerve across the transverse section.[4] The 30-degree test measures the change in thickness of the optic nerve when the patient moves the eye from primary gaze to 30 degrees of abduction. Initially, the maximum diameter is measured at the primary position and abduction at 30 degrees causes stretching of the nerve sheath and redistribution of cerebrospinal fluid in subarachnoid space and a net reduction of the optic nerve diameter. A reduction in the nerve measurement by more than 10–15% is considered a positive 30-degree test but variability due to operator-desired sensitivity and specificity cut-off values have to be taken into consideration.[4] Papilledema is optic disc edema due to increased intracranial pressure with subsequent increased accumulation of subarachnoid fluid giving a positive 30-degree test. In contrast, ODD does not cause an increase in subarachnoid fluid and thus the 30-degree test will be negative.[5] Elevation of the optic nerve is seen on B-scan ultrasound in both ODD and true papilledema and does not differentiate between the two possibilities.

The solution to Question 7 is A.

ODD can produce any form of nerve fiber layer visual field defect and, like glaucoma, an inferonasal or arcuate visual field defect is the most common (Fig. 2). Other visual field defects include altitudinal visual field defect, enlarged blind spot, and general constriction. Central or cecocentral scotomas are rare in ODD unless there is concomitant ischemic optic neuropathy or end-stage disease.[3] Central or cecocentral visual field defects or hemianopsia (bitemporal or homonymous) in patients with ODD should prompt further evaluation for alternative etiologies.

The solution to Question 8 is B.

The refractile bodies of ODD have an unusual internal property of autofluorescence that can be detected during the pre-injection stage of fundus fluorescein angiography. Hyperfluorescence can occur in both pseudopapilledema (staining) and true disc edema (leakage) on FFA. Papilledema shows a positive 30-degree test due to fluid in the sheath. The swelling of the optic disc head in true papilledema is due to accumulation of subarachnoid fluid in the optic disc head and produces elevation and obscuration of the peripapillary retinal nerve fiber layer that blurs the underlying retinal blood vessels as they cross the disc margin. Obligatory signs of increased intracranial pressure-related papilledema may also be present including retinal hemorrhages, cotton wool patches, and dilated retinal veins. These features are almost always absent in ODD, although some patients with ODD may have subretinal hemorrhages or an adjacent subretinal neovascular membrane that may make it difficult to differentiate. Blurred disc margins are seen in both true disc edema and ODD.

The solution to Question 9 is B.

Unfortunately, there is no effective treatment for ODD. However, visual field defects should be monitored for progression or for atypical findings that might prompt a search for alternative etiologies. Lee and Zimmerman described a progression of about 1.6% per year of visual field loss in patients with ODD.[9] In addition, as patients with ODD have glaucomatous-type visual field defects, superimposed glaucoma has to be considered in the differential diagnosis. The crowding of the optic disc head by ODD can mask glaucomatous cupping. In patients with borderline or elevated intraocular pressure (IOP) or progressive loss of visual field at a faster rate than expected by ODD, anti-glaucomatous eye drop could be considered. We tend to treat ocular hypertensive patients with ODD since ocular hypertension may exacerbate visual field loss in ODD. In one series of 103 eyes of 60 patients with ODD, 22 eyes were ocular hypertensive (mean IOP 27.1 ± 5 mmHg) and 81 were normotensive (mean IOP 15.7 ± 2.4 mmHg). Visual field loss was present in 20 of 22 (90.9%) ocular hypertensive eyes compared with only 54 of the 81 (66.7%) normotensive eyes. In this study, higher IOP was associated with a greater prevalence of visual field loss independent of age, sex, or whether the ODD is visible or buried.[10] Although there have been a few anecdotal reports of optic nerve sheath fenestration and radial optic neurotomy in patients with ODD, these remain unproven and not widely accepted treatment options.[11]

SUMMARY

Optic disc drusen (ODD) may be mistaken for true papilledema. Typically, the visual field defects of ODD are nerve fiber layer type deficits but central visual acuity is spared. B-scan ultrasound can detect calcified ODD but may miss non-calcified ODD. Likewise, CT scan can detect calcified ODD but the resolution and sensitivity of ultrasound is superior to CT. Some ODDs demonstrate autofluorescence and OCT has emerged as an additional imaging modality that might prove helpful in differentiating true edema from ODD.

REFERENCES

1. Khonsari RH, Wegener M, Leruez S, *et al.* (2010) Optic disc drusen or true papilledema? *Rev Neurol (Paris)* **166**:32–38.

2. Lam BL, Morais CG Jr, Pasol J. (2008) Drusen of the optic disc. *Curr Neurol Neurosci Rep* **8**:404–408.

3. Auw-Haedrich C, Staubach F, Witschel H. (2002) Optic disk drusen. *Surv Ophthalmol* **47**:515–532.

4. Atta HR. (1988) Imaging of the optic nerve with standardised echography. *Eye (Lond)* **2**:358–366.

5. Kurz-Levin mm, Landau K. (1999) A comparison of imaging techniques for diagnosing drusen of the optic nerve head. *Arch Ophthalmol* **117**:1045–1049.

6. Sarac O, Tasci YY, Gurdal C, Can I. (2012) Differentiation of optic disc edema from optic nerve head drusen with spectral-domain optical coherence tomography. *J Neuroophthalmol* **32**:207–211.

7. Mustonen E. (1983) Pseudopapilloedema with and without verified optic disc drusen. A clinical analysis II: visual fields. *Acta Ophthalmol (Copenh)* **61**:1057–1066.

8. Pollack IP, Becker B. (1962) Hyaline bodies (drusen) of the optic nerve. *Am J Ophthalmol* **54**:651–654.

9. Lee AG, Zimmerman MB. (2005) The rate of visual field loss in optic nerve head drusen. *Am J Ophthalmol* **139**:1062–1066.

10. Grippo T, Shihadeh W, Schargus M, *et al.* (2008) Optic nerve head drusen and visual field loss in normotensive and hypertensive eyes. *J Glaucoma* **17**:100–104.

11. Nentwich M, Remy M, Haritoglou C, Kampik A. (2011) Radial optic neurotomy to treat patients with visual field defects associated with optic nerve drusen. *Retina* **31**:612–615.

5

Pseudotumor Cerebri (Idiopathic Intracranial Hypertension)

Nagham Al-Zubidi MD, Jason Zhang BA, Arielle Spitze MD, Sushma Yalamanchili MD, and Andrew G. Lee MD

CASE

A 28-year-old female presented with acute binocular horizontal diplopia. She had no significant past medical history and her basal metabolic index (BMI) was 33. She complained of persistent and recurrent, severe, occipital headache, transient visual obscurations lasting 3–4 seconds at a time in both eyes (OU), pulse-synchronous tinnitus, as well as the binocular horizontal diplopia. She denied any photophobia, phonophobia, vertigo, or any other neurological symptoms. She was taking no medication and denied the use of medications causing increased intracranial pressure (ICP) (e.g., tetracycline, corticosteroids, vitamin A derivatives, lithium, nalidixic acid). The remainder of her past medical, surgical, medication, and social history was unremarkable.

On examination, her best-corrected visual acuity was 20/20 OU. The pupils measured 5 mm in the dark OU and 3 mm in the light OU, and there was no relative afferent pupillary defect (RAPD). Color vision plates were 14/14 OU. External examination, intraocular pressure measurements, and slit lamp biomicroscopy were normal OU. Motility exam showed a mild abduction deficit in the right eye (OD) with a 15-prism-diopter esotropia (ET) in primary position that increased to 25 PD ET in right gaze. Automated visual fields (Humphrey 24-2) showed enlarged blind spots OU with an inferior nasal step OD (see Fig. 5.1). Dilated funduscopic examination showed bilateral optic disc edema (i.e., papilledema) but the fundus examination was otherwise normal (see Fig. 5.2). Blood pressure measurement was normal. Magnetic resonance imaging (MRI) of the brain with and without gadolinium and magnetic resonance venography (MRV) showed no abnormalities except for a partially empty sella and bilateral flattening of the globe with cerebrospinal fluid (CSF) in the sheath consistent with increased intracranial pressure. Lumbar puncture showed an elevated opening pressure of 32 cm of water and normal CSF fluid contents. A presumptive diagnosis of pseudotumor cerebri (PTC) was made and the patient was started on acetazolamide. After 20 pounds of weight loss and three months of acetazolamide therapy the patient had complete resolution of all of her symptoms and signs of increased ICP.

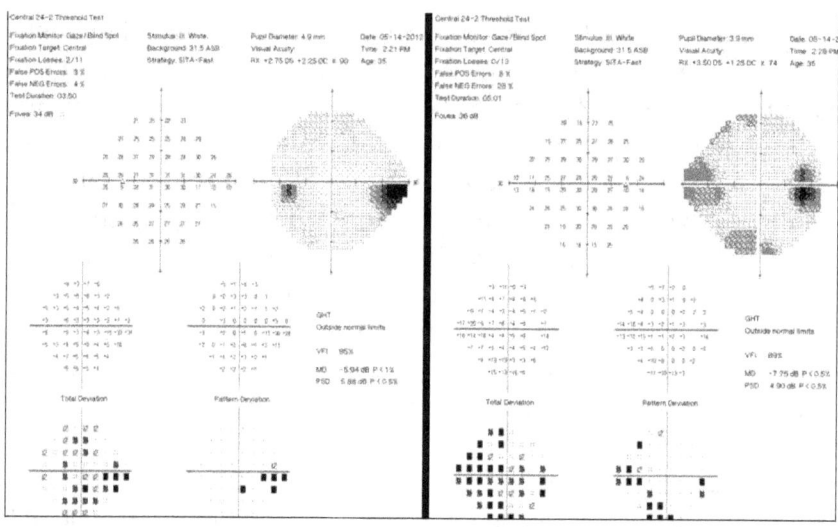

Fig. 5.1. Automated visual fields (Humphrey 24-2) showing enlarged blind spots OU with inferior nasal step OD.

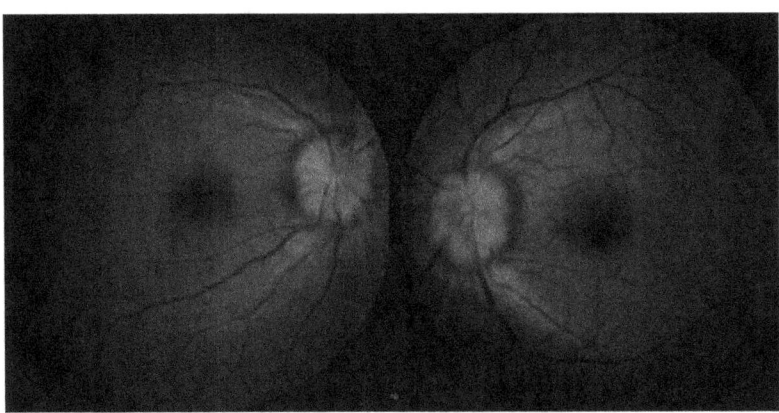

Fig. 5.2. Dilated funduscopic examination showing bilateral disc edema (papilledema).

Question 1	Question 2
Which of the following symptoms is most likely in typical idiopathic intracranial hypertension (IIH)?	**Which of the following signs is most consistent with IIH?**
A. Ataxia **B.** Paresthesias **C.** Diplopia **D.** Ptosis	**A.** Bilateral optic disc edema **B.** Bilateral central scotomas **C.** Incomitant right hypertropia **D.** Anterior or posterior uveitis
Question 3	Question 4
Which of the following patient demographics is most consistent with the diagnosis of IIH?	**Which of the following criteria is required in the modified Dandy criteria for IIH?**
A. 50-year-old thin female **B.** 25-year-old obese female **C.** 50-year-old thin male **D.** 25-year-old obese male	**A.** Elevated CSF protein **B.** Enlarged sella turcica **C.** Elevated opening pressure **D.** Bilateral optic disc edema

Question 5	Question 6
Which of the following is the neuroimaging study of choice for suspected IIH?	Which of the following treatments is considered to be first-line medical therapy for IIH?
A. Cranial MRI with/without contrast with MRV **B.** Cranial computed tomography (CT) scan and contrast CT angiography (CTA) **C.** MRA of the brain and orbits with contrast **D.** Contrast MRI of orbits with fat saturation	**A.** Topamax (topiramate) **B.** Prednisone **C.** Lasix (furosemide) **D.** Diamox (acetazolamide)
Question 7	**Question 8**
Which of the following is the next most appropriate step for severe, progressive visual field loss despite maximum medical therapy in IIH with a normal MRV?	Which of the following is the most common complication of optic nerve sheath fenestration?
A. Serial lumbar punctures **B.** Increase acetazolamide dose **C.** Venous sinus stenting **D.** Optic nerve sheath fenestration	**A.** Temporary diplopia **B.** Visual loss from central retinal artery occlusion (CRAO) **C.** Intracranial hemorrhage **D.** Slit ventricle syndrome

EXPLANATIONS

The solution to Question 1 is C.

The most common presenting symptom of idiopathic intracranial hypertension, or pseudotumor cerebri, is headache. The headache of IIH however is typically non-specific and varies in character, location, frequency, and severity.[1,2] The pain in IIH may also be facial or retrobulbar. Unfortunately other concomitant headache syndromes are common in patients with IIH including tension, migraine, and rebound headache. Other common presenting symptoms of IIH include unilateral or bilateral transient visual obscurations (seen in about two thirds of all IIH patients) that last for a few seconds at a time and pulse-synchronous tinnitus.[2] There also may be intermittent or constant binocular horizontal diplopia (typically due to a sixth nerve palsy as a non-localizing sign of increased ICP). Blurred vision due to IIH can be secondary to papilledema or macular edema, sub-retinal fluid, or hemorrhage. IIH requires that symptoms be confined to increased ICP and therefore other symptoms or signs not related to ICP are not consistent with IIH including cranial neuropathies (aside from cranial nerve VI palsy), hemisensory loss, hemiparesis, gait ataxia, ptosis, cerebellar, or reflex abnormalities.

The solution to Question 2 is A.

The most common sign in IIH is bilateral optic disc edema (i.e., papilledema) but is not required for the diagnosis.[3] Papilledema is often graded using the Frisen scale (from Grade 0 to Grade 5), and higher grades of papilledema and a longer duration of disc edema may be associated with a higher risk of permanent visual loss. Papilledema however may be asymmetric or even absent in IIH. In one study, it was found that up to 10% of patients with IIH had asymmetric papilledema.[4] Common visual field deficits in IIH include enlarged blind spots and any nerve fiber layer–type defect but central scotomas (from papillomacular bundle or macular involvement) would be an atypical and uncommon finding in IIH. Patients with a central scotoma should have a careful evaluation of the macula in IIH to exclude macular hemorrhage, edema, subretinal fluid, or exudates. Patients with an unexplained central visual acuity or visual field loss from IIH should have consideration for aggressive medical and surgical management including optic nerve sheath fenestration or cerebrospinal fluid shunting procedure. Although a non-localizing sixth nerve palsy and a secondary incomitant esotropia can occur in IIH, any other ocular deviation or other cranial neuropathy would be atypical and should prompt further evaluation. IIH is a non-inflammatory condition and the presence of anterior or posterior uveitis should raise the suspicion for an inflammatory etiology for the findings (e.g., sarcoidosis).

The solution to Question 3 is B.

Idiopathic intracranial hypertension is a disorder that primarily affects obese women of childbearing age.[1] In one prospective study of 50 IIH patients, 92% were women with a mean age of 31 years (range 11–58 years) and 94% were obese.[5] Although IIH can occur in males, children, the elderly, and patients with normal weight, the diagnosis should be scrutinized carefully in these populations. Particular attention should be devoted to excluding exogenous agents causing increased ICP such as steroids, growth hormone, tetracyclines (e.g., minocycline), vitamin A derivatives, and lithium.[1,6] In addition, certain systemic conditions including anemia, renal failure, Addison's disease, and systemic lupus erythematosus may also be associated with IIH.[7] Specific attention should be directed towards excluding cerebral venous sinus thrombosis and dural arteriovenous malformations as mimickers of IIH in atypical cases (e.g., thin, male, elderly) and an MRI with contrast MRV is generally recommended for the evaluation of papilledema in all patients but especially for patients who are not within the typical demographic for IIH.

The solution to Question 4 is C.

The modified Dandy criteria for the diagnosis of IIH include (1) symptoms and signs only due to increased ICP (e.g., headache, transient visual obscurations, pulse-synchronous tinnitus, papilledema, sixth nerve palsy, visual loss); (2) absence of any other neurological abnormalities or impaired consciousness; (3) elevated ICP with a normal CSF composition; (4) a neuroimaging study that excludes any etiology for the increased ICP (i.e., no venous sinus thrombosis); and (5) no secondary cause of intracranial hypertension.[8] The clinical evaluation of patients with IIH should include a complete history with particular attention paid to secondary causes of increased ICP including medications, hypercoagulable states, infectious processes, and systemic inflammatory processes. A typical ophthalmic examination should be supplemented with a formal visual field test, dilated funduscopic examination, and if possible baseline and follow-up optic nerve photographs. A lumbar puncture (with opening pressure, cell count and differential, glucose, and protein) is recommended after negative neuroimaging is performed. In patients with papilledema, checking the systemic blood pressure is important to exclude hypertensive optic neuropathy mimicking papilledema. Some authors have recommended complete blood count (CBC) testing, as severe anemia (typically iron deficiency) may be associated with IIH, but this is not a universally accepted recommendation.[9] While an elevated opening pressure is required for the diagnosis of IIH some patients have an artifactually normal or even low ICP measurement (e.g., after multiple attempts or a fluoroscopic lumbar puncture after failed conventional lumbar puncture). The MRI might show enlargement of the sella (i.e., empty sella) or CSF in the optic nerve sheath with posterior globe flattening as non-localizing radiographic signs of increased ICP. Papilledema, although common in IIH, is not required for the diagnosis according to the modified Dandy criteria and some patients with IIH have no papilledema.

The solution to Question 5 is A.

Magnetic resonance imaging of the brain with as well as without gadolinium with magnetic resonance venography is the imaging study of choice for IIH.[10] As noted above, several findings on MRI are highly suggestive but not diagnostic of increased ICP: (1) flattening of the posterior sclera (80%); (2) empty sella (70%); (3) distension of the perioptic subarachnoid space by CSF (50%); and (4) enhancement of the prelaminar optic nerve with gadolinium contrast (45%).[11] Cerebral venous sinus thrombosis (CVST) must be ruled out prior to the diagnosis of IIH and conventional cranial MRI may not show the lesion. While conventional MRI may sometimes detect CVST, both computed tomography venography (CTV) and MRV are significantly more sensitive for CVST. We highly recommend an MRV in addition to the cranial MRI even in patients who present with otherwise typical-appearing IIH.

The solution to Question 6 is D.

Although never proven by a randomized, controlled clinical trial, medical therapy with acetazolamide (Diamox) (typically initially 500 mg qd or bid with increasing dose to maximum tolerance up to 2–4 g as needed) is our recommended first-line agent in the treatment of symptomatic IIH.[12] However, an ongoing clinical trial is studying the efficacy of acetazolamide in IIH. Various case series have shown that acetazolamide is effective in symptomatic management and vision stabilization in up to 70% of patients with IIH. Although "sulfa allergy" and pregnancy should prompt caution in the use of acetazolamide, there is limited evidence to support not using acetazolamide in patients with non-anaphylactic allergic or adverse reactions to "sulfa"-containing agents, and pregnant patients (especially in the third trimester) might still benefit from medical treatment. Consultation with the treating obstetrician should be performed prior to treatment of IIH patients who are pregnant but in general the evaluation and management of pregnant and non-pregnant patients with IIH is the same. Gadolinium and acetazolamide are FDA class C agents and a risk-benefit decision need to be made on an individual basis for their use in pregnant patients with IIH. In patients on acetazolamide, although serum electrolytes could be checked and followed, most clinicians simply warn the patient and the primary physician about the potential side effects, including the risk of metabolic acidosis and kidney stones without routine serial electrolyte testing in low-risk patients. Furosemide (20–40 mg per day for adults) is often considered a second-line therapy for IIH but has been used effectively in combination with acetazolamide. Thiazide diuretics have yet to show any proven benefit in patients with IIH but might be considered. Topiramate, an anti-epileptic medication with carbonic anhydrase inhibition properties similar in mechanism to that of acetazolamide, is also often used as an alternative therapy in patients who cannot tolerate Diamox.[13] Clinicians should be aware that topiramate may cause ocular side effects including angle closure glaucoma and induced myopia. Long-term medical therapy should always be conducted in conjunction with dietary and behavioral modifications (weight loss, exercise, etc.).

The solution to Question 7 is D.

The primary indications for surgical intervention in patients with IIH are (1) a progressive visual field defect or intractable headache despite maximum medical therapy; (2) patients who are non-compliant or intolerant to treatment.[14] The two main surgical interventions in patients with PTC are cerebrospinal fluid shunting procedures (such as a ventriculoperitoneal or lumboperitoneal shunt) and optic nerve sheath fenestration (ONSF). Although serial lumbar punctures may be useful in rare circumstances to control ICP prior to surgery or as a temporizing therapy (e.g., pregnant patient avoiding medical or surgical treatment) we generally advise against serial lumbar punctures in IIH. The CSF also reforms very quickly after a lumbar puncture and thus there is little theoretical reason for this treatment to work on a long-term basis. In addition, serial lumbar punctures are uncomfortable and can result in complications, including low-pressure headache, CSF leak, and CSF infection. A lumbar drain however might be a reasonable alternative temporizing measure for acute, fulminant IIH with visual loss prior to admission and consideration for definitive surgical treatment of papilledema. Cerebral venous stenting[15] is a relatively new and still controversial procedure based on observations that many IIH patients have stenosis of the transverse venous sinus. Although in the future stenting procedures for venous sinus stenosis in IIH might be proven useful it does not at this time have any proven role in patients with a normal MRV. The first-line surgical intervention for visual loss despite maximum medical therapy in our practice is optic nerve sheath fenestration but CSF shunting may be necessary at institutions where ONSF is not available or perhaps for patients who wish to undergo only a single surgery or who have concomitant intractable headache as the indication for surgery. Bariatric surgery in markedly obese patients might also be a useful surgical intervention but takes time to reach effect.

The solution to Question 8 is A.

Temporary diplopia is one of the most common complications of ONSF and may be the result of edema or less commonly direct trauma to the extraocular muscles, nerves, or blood supply.[16] Transient diplopia occurs in up to 29–35% of cases following ONSF. Other common complications of ONSF include pupillary dysfunction (11%) and temporary decreased visual acuity (11%). Permanent and severe visual loss (e.g., CRAO or optic nerve damage) fortunately are rare after ONSF. Both CSF shunting procedures and ONSF have various other surgical and anesthesia-related potential complications, though ONSF is in general considered a safer and less invasive procedure. In one of the largest case series published to date, Banta and Farris reported that out of 158 operations, 94% reported stabilized or improved visual acuity and 88% reported stabilized or improved visual fields.[17] In smaller case series, ONSF generally has better outcomes in patients with a shorter duration of visual disturbance and less severe symptoms. ONSF might also be the preferred surgical modality in children. Eyes that undergo ONSF often have a recurrence of the initial symptoms (~2–32%) and may require repeat surgery.

Although CSF shunting procedures have a higher success rate, the incidence of complications is significantly higher than that of ONSF.[18,19] Shunt failure occurs in 50–80% of patients, often requiring multiple revisions. Other common complications include shunt infection, abdominal pain, and other postoperative complications. Tonsillar herniation and slit ventricle syndrome are rare complications of CSF shunts and unfortunately in at least one series the inpatient mortality for CSF shunting was as high as 0.9% for ventriculoperitoneal shunting and 0.3% for lumboperitoneal shunting. In addition, in patients with venous sinus thrombosis and dural arteriovenous fistula mimicking IIH as the cause of increased ICP and papilledema, lumboperitoneal shunting might cause more harm than good and in general in this clinical setting we recommend ONSF rather than lumboperitoneal shunting.

SUMMARY

Idiopathic intracranial hypertension is characterized by increased ICP of undetermined cause and is a diagnosis of exclusion. IIH is characterized clinically by headache, pulse-synchronous tinnitus, diplopia, transient visual obscurations, and blurred vision. Ophthalmological findings often include bilateral papilledema leading to the common visual field defect or enlarged blind spots but any nerve fiber layer defect can be associated with IIH and untreated, undertreated, or acute, fulminant IIH can lead to permanent blindness in one or both eyes. The disorder is predominantly seen in women of childbearing age and may be associated with a history of recent weight gain. The diagnostic criteria for IIH based upon the modified Dandy criteria include (1) symptoms and signs of increased intracranial pressure; (2) absence of any other neurological abnormalities or impaired consciousness except for sixth nerve palsy; (3) elevated intracranial pressure with a normal cerebrospinal fluid composition; (4) a neuroimaging study that excludes any etiology for the increased intracranial pressure (typically an MRI with and without contrast with a post-contrast MRV); and (5) no secondary cause of intracranial hypertension. In addition to imaging, systemic blood pressure readings, an ophthalmologic examination, formal visual field testing, and a lumbar puncture are typically necessary in the diagnostic evaluation of papilledema. Medical therapy is typically initiated with acetazolamide, although furosemide and topiramate may be effective second-line or adjuvant agents as well. If the visual loss or headache fails to resolve despite maximum medical therapy, then surgical options include optic nerve sheath fenestration (especially for papilledema-related visual loss) and various cerebrospinal fluid shunting procedures could be considered. A lumbar drain might be a reasonable temporizing measure for acute, fulminant IIH with visual loss during the hospital admission and in preparation for definitive surgical treatment of papilledema-related visual loss. Cerebral venous sinus stenting remains controversial but may prove to be another potential therapy for IIH in patients with venous sinus stenosis.

REFERENCES

1. Wall M. (2010) Idiopathic intracranial hypertension. *Neurol Clin* **28**:593–617.
2. Wall M. (1990) The headache profile of idiopathic intracranial hypertension. *Cephalalgia* **10**:331–335.
3. Digre KB, Nakamoto BK,Warner JE, *et al.* (2009) A comparison of idiopathic intracranial hypertension with and without papilledema. *Headache* **49**: 185–193.
4. Wall M, White WN 2nd. (1998) Asymmetric papilledema in idiopathic intracranial hypertension: prospective interocular comparison of sensory visual function. *Invest Ophthalmol Vis Sci* **39**(1):134–142.
5. Wall M, George D. (1991) Idiopathic intracranial hypertension. A prospective study of 50 patients. *Brain* **114**:155–180.
6. Friedman DI. (2005) Medication-induced intracranial hypertension in dermatology. *Am J Clin Dermatol* **6**:29–37.
7. Barahona-Hernando R, Rios-Blanco JJ, Mendez-Meson I, *et al.* (2009) Idiopathic intracranial hypertension and systemic lupus erythematosus: a case report and review of the literature. *Lupus* **18**:1121–1123.
8. Friedman DI, Jacobson DM. (2002) Diagnostic criteria for idiopathic intracranial hypertension. *Neurology* **59**:1492–1495.
9. Mollan SP, Ball AK, Sinclair AJ, *et al.* (2009) Idiopathic intracranial hypertension associated with iron deficiency anaemia: a lesson for management. *Eur Neurol* **62**:105–108.
10. Brodsky MC, Vaphiades M. (1998) Magnetic resonance imaging in pseudotumor cerebri. *Ophthalmology* **105**:1686–1693.
11. Degnan AJ, Levy LM. (2011) Pseudotumor cerebri: brief review of clinical syndrome and imaging findings. *AJNR Am J Neuroradiol* **32**:1986–1993.
12. Biousse V, Bruce BB, Newman NJ. (2012) Update on the pathophysiology and management of idiopathic intracranial hypertension. *J Neurol Neurosurg Psychiatry* **83**:488–494.
13. Celebisoy N, Gokcay F, Sirin H, Akyurekli O. (2007) Treatment of idiopathic intra-cranial hypertension: topiramate vs. acetazolamide, an open-label study. *Acta Neuro Scand* **116**:322–327.
14. Uretsky S. (2009) Surgical interventions for idiopathic intracranial hypertension. *Curr Opin Ophthalmol* **20**:451–455.
15. Bussiere M, Falero R, Nicolle D, *et al.* (2010) Unilateral transverse sinus stenting of patients with idiopathic intracranial hypertension. *AJNR Am J Neuroradiol* **31**:645–650.
16. Plotnik JL, Kosmorsky GS. (1993) Operative complications of optic nerve sheath decompression. *Ophthalmology* **100**:683–690.
17. Banta JT, Farris BK. (2000) Pseudotumor cerebri and optic nerve sheath decompression. *Ophthalmology* **107**:1907–1912.

18. Spitze A, Malik A, Al-Zubidi N, *et al.* (2013) Optic nerve sheath fenestration vs cerebrospinal diversion procedures: what is the preferred surgical procedure for the treatment of idiopathic intracranial hypertension failing maximum medical therapy? *J Neuroophthalmol* **33**:183–188.
19. Ulivieri S, Oliveri G, Georgantzinou M, *et al.* (2009) Long-term effectiveness of lumboperitoneal-regulated shunt system for idiopathic intracranial hypertension. *J Neurosurg Sci* **53**:107–111.

6

Non-arteritic Anterior Ischemic Optic Neuropathy (NAION)

Arielle Spitze MD, Christopher Pruet MD, Nagham Al-Zubidi MD, Sushma Yalamanchili MD, and Andrew G. Lee MD

CASE

A 65-year-old male presented with acute, painless vision loss in the lower portion of his left eye (OS) for one day. Past medical history was significant for hypertension, hyperlipidemia, and coronary artery disease with previous coronary artery stenting. Significant medications included aspirin and clopidogrel (Plavix). He smoked one pack of cigarettes per day for many years. He denied jaw claudication, scalp pain, headache, fever, chills, or malaise and had no history of obstructive sleep apnea. He was not using any phosphodiesterase inhibitors (erectile dysfunction medications). External examination was negative for temporal nodularity or scalp tenderness. Visual acuity was 20/20 in the right eye (OD) and 20/400 OS. The pupils measured 4 mm in the dark and 2 mm in the light in both eyes (OU), but there was a relative afferent pupillary defect (RAPD) OS. The remainder of the anterior segment examination was within normal limits. Automated visual field testing (Humphrey 24-2) was normal OD but showed a dense inferior arcuate field defect OS (Fig. 6.1). Dilated fundus examination OD was normal and showed a cup-to-disc ratio of 0.1 (Fig. 6.2). There was superior (sectoral) disc edema OS (Fig. 6.3) that resolved over time to residual sectoral optic atrophy OS. Optical coherence tomography (OCT) of the optic nerve OS showed a thinned superior nerve fiber layer (Fig. 6.4) six months later. Laboratory workup at the time of

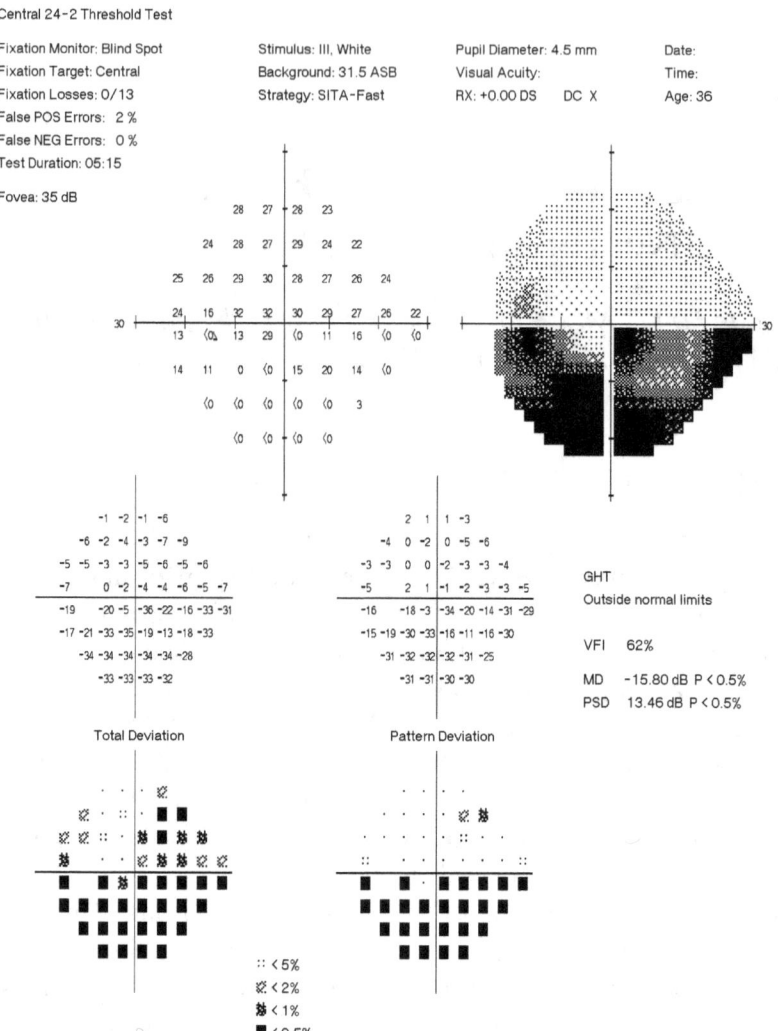

Fig. 6.1. Visual field demonstrating a dense inferior arcuate field defect in the left eye.

presentation revealed a normal erythrocyte sedimentation rate (ESR) and C-reactive protein (CRP) level. General physical examination was normal and carotid Doppler testing performed by internal medicine showed less than 40% stenosis bilaterally.

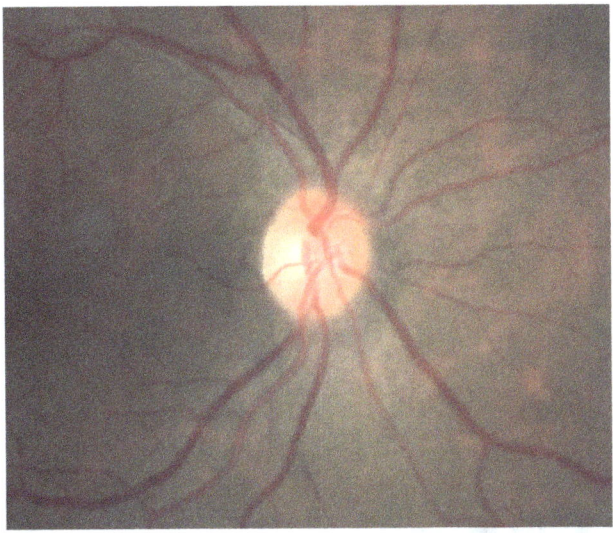

Fig. 6.2. Optic nerve photo of the non-involved (right) eye showing a small cup-to-disc ratio.

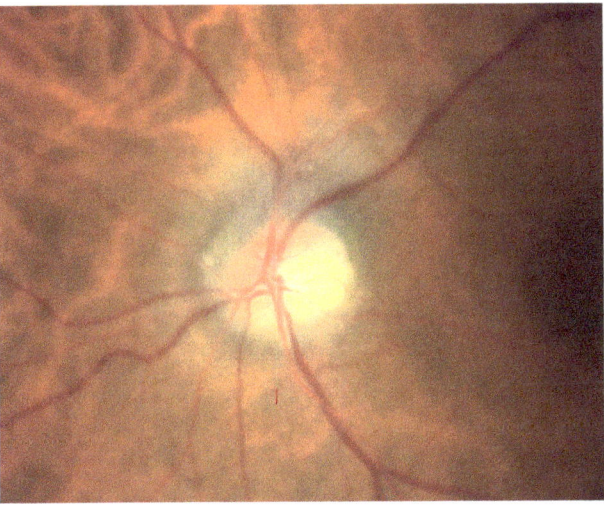

Fig. 6.3. Optic nerve photo of the involved (left) eye showing superior, sectoral disc edema with blurring of the superior disc margin vessels.

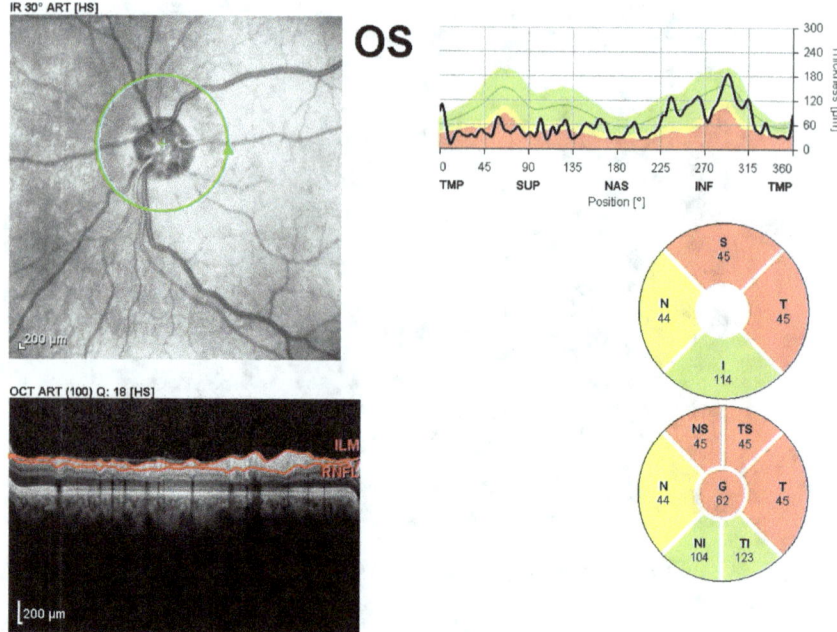

Fig. 6.4. OCT of the left optic nerve six months after initial presentation, showing superior thinning of the nerve fiber layer.

Question 1	Question 2
Which of the following symptoms is most consistent with the visual loss experienced by a patient with NAION?	Which of the following is most helpful in differentiating arteritic anterior ischemic optic neuropathy (A-AION, or giant cell arteritis) from NAION?
A. Painful B. Acute C. Bilateral D. Progressive	A. Small cup-to-disc ratio B. Older-age population C. Type of visual field loss D. Pallid disc edema

Question 3	Question 4
Which of the following is a risk factor for the development of NAION?	**According to the Ischemic Optic Neuropathy Decompression Trial (IONDT), which of the following was the outcome in patients who were treated with surgery compared with observation for NAION?**
A. Large cup-to-disc ratio **B.** Nocturnal hypertension **C.** Dialysis-dependent renal disease **D.** Aspirin or other anti-platelet use	**A.** No improvement in either arm of study **B.** More patients in the surgical arm had worsened vision of three lines or more **C.** Modest improvement favoring surgical arm **D.** Marked improvement favoring surgical arm
Question 5	Question 6
Which of the following is the best estimated risk of having recurrent NAION in the same eye after one episode of NAION?	**What is the risk of having NAION occur in the fellow eye after one eye is affected with NAION?**
A. < 5% **B.** 15% **C.** 25% **D.** 78%	**A.** < 5% **B.** 15% **C.** 25% **D.** 78%
Question 7	Question 8
Which of the following treatment options for NAION showed benefit in a patient choice methodology study?	**According to the IONDT, which of the following best represents the percentage of patients with NAION who will experience spontaneous improvement in vision of three lines or more?**
A. Intravitreal anti-VEGF treatment **B.** Optic nerve sheath decompression **C.** Oral prednisone **D.** Tissue plasminogen activator	**A.** 2% **B.** 22% **C.** 42% **D.** 62%

EXPLANATIONS

The solution to Question 1 is B.

The distinctive symptoms of NAION are acute-onset (often noted upon awakening), monocular, and painless visual acuity or visual field loss. The presumed mechanism of NAION is ischemia to the anterior portion of the optic nerve.[1–5] Although unproven, one hypothesis is that NAION is the result of hypoperfusion of the optic nerve with secondary swelling of the anterior optic nerve that might produce a compartment syndrome, resulting in a vicious cycle of further vascular compromise and secondary ischemia.[6,7] Thus, a small cup-to-disc ratio (crowded optic nerve head) has been hypothesized to be a predisposing risk factor for NAION (the "disc at risk"). The classically affected superotemporal nerve fibers result in a corresponding inferonasal field defect in typical NAION, but any part of the optic nerve head can be involved.[8] If the ischemia involves the papillomacular bundle, central visual acuity can be decreased, but this occurs in less than half of patients with NAION.[8] Although NAION-related visual field loss normally respects the horizontal meridian (nerve fiber layer), respect of the vertical meridian would be more suggestive of a process involving the intracranial portion of the optic nerve in unilateral cases (junctional) or a chiasmal/retrochiasmal etiology if the vision loss respected the vertical meridian bilaterally. Bilateral NAION can occur simultaneously, but this is an atypical presentation and usually bilateral cases of NAION are sequential and non-simultaneous. Episodes can often be separated by several months to years. Pain on eye movement is more common in optic neuritis and typically does not occur in NAION, but could be present in a minority of patients. Progression can occur in NAION, but is uncommon.

The solution to Question 2 is D.

Giant cell arteritis (GCA) most commonly affects the posterior ciliary arteries, but can also affect the central retinal artery (CRAO) or ophthalmic artery.[1] GCA is a systemic vasculitis and unlike NAION may involve the cilioretinal artery,[9–12] central retinal artery,[12] or choroidal circulation.[9]

Choroidal involvement may be seen as choroidal hypoperfusion on fluorescein angiography. If GCA is suspected, an ESR and CRP are non-specific inflammatory markers that are sensitive for GCA but not specific.[13] A temporal artery biopsy is the diagnostic gold standard for GCA.[13] Although a small cup-to-disc ratio (i.e., the "disc at risk" for NAION) is suggestive of NAION, a small cup can occur in patients with GCA. In contrast, however, the presence of a large cup-to-disc ratio makes the diagnosis of NAION less likely and should raise the suspicion for GCA. In addition, the disc in NAION is typically hyperemic with sectoral or diffuse optic disc edema. Conversely, pallid edema (ischemic infarction of the disc) in the acute setting is a red flag for GCA. The absence of pallid edema, however, does not exclude GCA. In NAION, the anterior optic nerve is affected and thus disc edema must be present at onset. In GCA, the disc is typically swollen (A-AION) but may be normal in appearance in posterior ION (PION). The presence of PION is highly suggestive of GCA over non-arteritic mechanisms. Although younger patients (< 50 years old) do not typically develop GCA, both NAION and GCA can occur in older patients with or without concomitant vasculopathic risk factors. Thus, although a younger age (< 50 years) suggests NAION over A-AION and an older age should raise suspicion for GCA, older age alone does not differentiate the two.

Many varieties of nerve fiber layer defects or central visual field defects can occur in both A-AION and NAION, so the type and severity of the visual field defect cannot be used to differentiate between the two mechanisms. Although the visual loss in A-AION tends to be more severe than NAION, either condition can present with any severity of visual loss.[14] Patients with light perception or no light perception vision, with bilateral simultaneous onset, or progression, however, are more likely to be harboring GCA.

The solution to Question 3 is C.

There are multiple proposed risk factors for NAION and it is likely that the disorder is multifactorial. Patients with NAION can have both predisposing and precipitating factors for visual loss. The conditions which might increase the risk of NAION include vasculopathic conditions (e.g., hypertension, diabetes mellitus, heart disease, hyperlipidemia, or atherosclerosis[2,15–18]), poor oxygen-carrying capacity (smoking, obstructive sleep apnea,[2,19–21] anemia[22]), and physiologic ocular variations (small cup-to-disc ratio[14,23] or increased intraocular pressure[24]).

Nocturnal hypotension (rather than nocturnal hypertension)[25–28] has been proposed as a possible precipitating mechanism for NAION, especially in patients with predisposing vasculopathic risk factors (including hypertension). Some authors have advised patients with NAION to take their antihypertensive medications in the morning to avoid the potential for nocturnal hypotension. Although aspirin has not been proven to improve function in affected eyes, it remains controversial whether aspirin imparts any influence on occurrence in the fellow eye. Nevertheless, many clinicians offer aspirin or antiplatelet therapy to patients with NAION as a preventative measure, mostly because they harbor vasculopathic risk factors that could lead to cardiac or neurologic ischemic events.

Patients with end-stage renal disease and on dialysis may be at particular risk for NAION because they have multiple factors contributing to hypoperfusion and secondary risk factors for NAION (e.g., anemia, hypotension, fluid shifts, decreased oxygen-carrying capacity, hypertension, diabetes, sleep apnea).

The solution to Question 4 is B.

In the IONDT, patients assigned to optic nerve sheath decompression surgery (ONDS) did no better when compared with patients assigned to careful follow-up (32.6% of the ONDS group improved by three or more lines of visual acuity at six months, compared with 42.7% of the controls). The odds ratio (OR) for three or more lines better visual acuity, adjusted for baseline visual acuity and diabetes, was 0.74 (95% CI, 0.39–1.38). In addition, patients receiving surgery had a significantly greater risk of losing three or more lines of vision at six months (23.9% compared with 12.4% of the controls). The six-month adjusted OR for three or more lines worsening visual acuity was 1.96 (95% CI, 0.87–4.41). There was also no difference in treatment effect for patients with progressive NAION. Thus, the IONDT concluded that ONDS for NAION is not effective, may be harmful, and should be abandoned.[29,30] A clinical alert to this effect was issued on January 3, 1995, by the National Eye Institute and the IONDT to all ophthalmologists, neuro-ophthalmologists, and neurologists.

The solution to Question 5 is A.

If the crowded optic disc hypothesis for NAION is true, then because a portion of the nerve fiber layer is damaged after the initial episode of NAION, there is additional space created for existing nerve fibers to expand should a second vascular insult occur again at the disc head. This has led some authors to speculate that this is the reason for the very low risk of recurrence of NAION in the same eye (< 5%).[30] Recurrent NAION in the same eye should raise a red flag that the diagnosis of NAION may not be correct, or perhaps that an underlying risk factor remains undiagnosed or untreated.

The solution to Question 6 is B.

The risk of NAION to the fellow eye in the IONDT was about 15%. Presumably, because the same predisposing risk factors are often present in the same patient and thus in both eyes, the fellow eye has about a 15% risk of being affected by NAION.[31] Risk factors in one study for developing NAION in the fellow eye included poor visual acuity in the affected eye and diabetes mellitus, but not age, gender, or smoking history. Aspirin use has shown conflicting data for reducing occurrence in the fellow eye, but is often recommended by clinicians for reducing other cardiovascular events.[32,33]

The solution to Question 7 is C.

Prednisone in the literature has shown variable and sometimes conflicting results for the treatment of NAION. Hayreh *et al.* found improvement in visual acuity in 69.8% ($n = 236$) of oral prednisone–treated patients versus improvement in only 40.5% ($n = 301$) of untreated patients in a non-blinded prospective patient choice methodology study ($p = 0.001$).[34] In contrast, Rebolleda *et al.* found no statistically significant benefit from using oral prednisone treatment in visual acuity, median deviation on Humphrey visual fields, or retinal nerve fiber layer thickness (treatment $n = 9$, control $n = 27$) in NAION.[35] Thus, because conflict remains concerning the use of oral corticosteroids in acute NAION,[36,37] decisions to treat with oral prednisone should be made on a case-by-case basis.

The IONDT noted that ONDS was not effective and might be harmful in NAION.[29,30] Hyperbaric oxygen therapy has also been used in some reports without much success.[37] Aspirin may have some ability to decrease the risk of NAION occurrence in the fellow eye (conflicting data),[32,33] but has not been shown to be efficacious in the affected eye.[39] Tissue plasminogen activator (TPA) has not been studied in NAION, but because the disease is thought to be caused by small vessel ischemic hypoperfusion and not thromboembolic or thrombotic disease, TPA would not likely be beneficial. Erythropoietin has been investigated in NAION and has shown some promise in small series, but anti-vascular endothelial growth factors have had limited effect in only a handful of studies, and have not been confirmed with randomized controlled trials. Until a randomized controlled clinical trial of steroids in NAION is performed, it is our practice to alert patients to the existence of the Hayreh patient choice methodology study and to offer steroids as an option, but we discourage treatment in patients with significant potential risk for steroids (e.g., uncontrolled diabetes).

The solution to Question 8 is C.

Approximately 42% of patients with NAION in the IONDT experienced some spontaneous improvement in visual acuity (three lines or more) after their initial ischemic insult.[29,30,34] These changes generally stabilize over six months from the initial time of insult.[39]

SUMMARY

NAION typically presents as an acute, monocular, painless loss of vision in a vasculopathic older-aged patient with a crowded, small optic disc (i.e., the structural "disc at risk"). The proposed risk factors for developing NAION include vasculopathic (diabetes, hypertension, hyperlipidemia, atherosclerosis, etc.), hypoxic (anemia, low oxygen tension), and ocular (small cup-to-disc ratio, increased intraocular pressure) factors. Proposed precipitating events can include nocturnal hypotension, shock, acute hemorrhage, acute hypoxemia, or acutely increased intraocular pressure. The typical symptoms of NAION include acute painless visual loss typically with inferonasal visual field defects, but roughly 50% of NAION events involve the central visual field. The signs of NAION include a relative afferent pupillary defect in the affected eye and diffuse or sectoral disc edema. Acute treatment may involve oral prednisone, although this is still controversial and treatment decisions should be made on an individual basis. Management should focus on controlling predisposing or precipitating vasculopathic risk factors. Despite this, up to 5% of patients will have a recurrence in the same eye, and up to 15% may develop NAION in the fellow eye.

REFERENCES

1. Hayreh SS. (2009) Ischemic optic neuropathy. *Prog Retin Eye Res* **28**:34–62.
2. Hayreh SS. (1996) Acute ischemic disorders of the optic nerve: pathogenesis, clinical manifestations, and management. *Ophthalmol Clin N Am* **9**:407–442.
3. Hayreh SS. (1974) Anterior ischaemic optic neuropathy. I. Terminology and pathogenesis. *Br J Ophthalmol* **58**:955–963.
4. Hayreh SS. (1981) Anterior ischemic optic neuropathy. *Arch Neurol* **38**: 675–678.
5. Hayreh SS. (1985) Inter-individual variation in blood supply of the optic nerve head. Its importance in various ischemic disorders of the optic nerve head, and glaucoma, low-tension glaucoma and allied disorders. *Doc Ophthalmol* **59**:217–246.
6. Beck RW, Servais GE, Hayreh SS. (1987) Anterior ischemic optic neuropathy. IX. Cup-to-disc ratio and its role in pathogenesis. *Ophthalmology* **94**:1503–1508.

7. Hayreh SS, Zimmerman MB. (2008) Nonarteritic anterior ischemic optic neuropathy: refractive error and its relationship to cup/disc ratio. *Ophthalmology* **115**:2275–2281.

8. Hayreh SS, Zimmerman B. (2005) Visual field abnormalities in nonarteritic anterior ischemic optic neuropathy: their pattern and prevalence at initial examination. *Arch Ophthalmol* **123**:1554–1562.

9. Hayreh SS. (1974) Anterior ischaemic optic neuropathy. II. Fundus on ophthalmoscopy and fluorescein angiography. *Br J Ophthalmol* **58**:964–980.

10. Hayreh SS. (1978) Ischemic optic neuropathy. *Int Ophthalmol* **1**:9–18.

11. Hayreh SS. (1990) Anterior ischaemic optic neuropathy differentiation of arteritic from non-arteritic type and its management. *Eye* **4**:25–41.

12. Hayreh SS, Podhajsky PA, Zimmerman B. (1998) Ocular manifestations of giant cell arteritis. *Am J Ophthalmol* **125**:509–520.

13. Hayreh SS, Podhajsky PA, Raman R, Zimmerman B. (1997) Giant cell arteritis: validity and reliability of various diagnostic criteria. *Am J Ophthalmol* **123**:285–296.

14. Hayreh SS, Zimmerman MB. (2008) Non-arteritic anterior ischemic optic neuropathy: role of systemic corticosteroid therapy. *Graefes Arch Clin Exp Ophthalmol* **246**:1029–1046.

15. Repka MX, Savino PJ, Schatz NJ, Sergott RC. (1983) Clinical profile and long-term implications of anterior ischemic optic neuropathy. *Am J Ophthalmol* **96**:478–483.

16. Guyer DR, Miller NR, Auer CL, Fine SL. (1985) The risk of cerebrovascular and cardiovascular disease in patients with anterior ischemic optic neuropathy. *Arch Ophthalmol* **103**:1136–1142.

17. Hayreh SS, Joos KM, Podhajsky PA, Long CR. (1994) Systemic diseases associated with nonarteritic anterior ischemic optic neuropathy. *Am J Ophthalmol* **118**:766–780.

18. Jacobson DM, Vierkant RA, Belongia EA. (1997) Nonarteritic anterior ischemic optic neuropathy: a case-control study of potential risk factors. *Arch Ophthalmol* **115**:1403–1407.

19. Mojon DS, Hedges TR 3rd, Ehrenberg B, *et al.* (2002) Association between sleep apnea syndrome and nonarteritic anterior ischemic optic neuropathy. *Arch Ophthalmol* **120**:601–605.

20. Palombi K, Renard E, Levy P, *et al.* (2006) Non-arteritic anterior ischaemic optic neuropathy is nearly systematically associated with obstructive sleep apnoea. *Br J Ophthalmol* **90**:879–882.

21. Li J, McGwin G Jr, Vaphiades MS, Owsley C. (2007) Non-arteritic anterior ischaemic optic neuropathy and presumed sleep apnoea syndrome screened by the sleep apnea scale of the sleep disorders questionnaire (SA-SDQ). *Br J Ophthalmol* **91**:1524–1527.

22. Hayreh SS. (1987) Anterior ischemic optic neuropathy. VIII. Clinical features and pathogenesis of post-hemorrhagic amaurosis. *Ophthalmology* **94**:1488–1502.

23. Beck RW, Servais GE, Hayreh SS. (1987) Anterior ischemic optic neuropathy. IX. Cup-to-disc ratio and its role in pathogenesis. *Ophthalmology* **94**:1503–1508.

24. Hayreh SS. (1980) Anterior ischemic optic neuropathy. IV. Occurrence after cataract extraction. *Arch Ophthalmol* **98**:1410–1416.

25. Hayreh SS, Zimmerman MB, Podhajsky P, Alward WLM. (1994) Nocturnal arterial hypotension and its role in optic nerve head and ocular ischemic disorders. *Am J Ophthalmol* **117**:603–624.

26. Hayreh SS, Podhajsky PA, Zimmerman B. (1997) Nonarteritic anterior ischemic optic neuropathy: time of onset of visual loss. *Am J Ophthalmol* **124**:641–647.

27. Hayreh SS, Podhajsky P, Zimmerman MB. (1999) Role of nocturnal arterial hypotension in optic nerve head ischemic disorders. *Ophthalmologica* **213**:76–96.

28. Hayreh SS, Servais GE, Virdi PS. (1986) Fundus lesions in malignant hypertension. V. Hypertensive optic neuropathy. *Ophthalmology* **93**:74–87.

29. Ischemic Optic Neuropathy Decompression Trial: twenty-four-month update. (2000) *Arch Ophthalmol* **118**:793–798.

30. The Ischemic Optic Neuropathy Decompression Trial Research Group. (1995) Optic nerve decompression surgery for nonarteritic anterior ischemic optic neuropathy (NAION) is not effective and may be harmful. *JAMA* **273**:625–632.

31. Luneau K, Newman NJ, Biousse V. (2008) Ischemic optic neuropathies. *Neurologist* **14**:341–354.

32. Salomon O, Huna-Baron R, Steinberg DM, *et al.* (1999) Role of aspirin in reducing the frequency of second eye involvement in patients with non-arteritic anterior ischaemic optic neuropathy. *Eye* **13**:357–359.

33. Newman NJ, Scherer R, Langenberg P, *et al.* (2002) The fellow eye in NAION: report from the ischemic optic neuropathy decompression trial follow-up study. *Am J Ophthalmol* **134**:317–328.

34. Hayreh SS. (2010) Non-arteritic anterior ischemic optic neuropathy: role of systemic corticosteroid therapy. *Surv Ophthalmol* **55**:399–400; author reply 400–401.

35. Rebolleda G, Perez-Lopez M, Casas-Llera P, *et al.* (2013) Visual and anatomical outcomes of non-arteritic anterior ischemic optic neuropathy with high-dose systemic corticosteroids. *Graefes Arch Clin Exp Ophthalmol* **251**:255–260.

36. Atkins EJ, Bruce BB, Newman NJ, Biousse V. (2010) Treatment of nonarteritic anterior ischemic optic neuropathy. *Surv Ophthalmol* **55**:47–63.

37. Lee AG, Biousse V. (2010) Should steroids be offered to patients with nonarteritic anterior ischemic optic neuropathy? *J Neuroophthalmol* **30**:193–198.

38. Arnold AC, Levin LA. (2002) Treatment of ischemic optic neuropathy. *Semin Ophthalmol* **17**:39–46.

39. Botelho PJ, Johnson LN, Arnold AC. (1996) The effect of aspirin on the visual outcome of nonarteritic anterior ischemic optic neuropathy. *Am J Ophthalmol* **121**:450–451.

40. Hayreh SS, Zimmerman MB. (2008) Nonarteritic anterior ischemic optic neuropathy: natural history of visual outcome. *Ophthalmology* **115**:298–305e2.

7

Arteritic Anterior Ischemic Optic Neuropathy (A-AION)

Arielle Spitze MD, Claudia G. Hooten MD, Nagham Al-Zubidi MD, Sushma Yalamanchili MD, and Andrew G. Lee MD

CASE

A 77-year-old man presented with acute, painless, decreased vision in the right eye (OD) for one day. Past medical history was significant for hypertension. He had a few recent episodes of transient blackouts of vision OD, increased generalized fatigue, a right-sided headache with associated tenderness of the right temple, and pain while chewing his food for the past few weeks. He denied recent trauma, neck pain, or any other significant symptoms. On external examination, there was temporal tenderness on the right and the temporal artery was nodular to palpation. Best-corrected visual acuity was 20/400 OD and 20/40 in the left eye (OS). Pupils measured 4 mm in the dark and 2 mm in the light in both eyes (OU) with a right relative afferent pupillary defect. Extraocular motility was full and the eyes were orthotropic in all positions of gaze. Humphrey visual field (24-2) using a stimulus V showed general depression OD and scattered non-specific defects using a stimulus III OS. Anterior segment exam was within normal limits OU. Dilated fundus examination revealed pallid disc edema OD (see Fig. 7.1). The left fundus examination was unremarkable. Fluorescein angiography showed patchy delayed choroidal hypoperfusion OD and normal retinal and choroidal perfusion OS. Erythrocyte sedimentation rate (ESR) was elevated at 73 mm/hr and a C-reactive protein (CRP) was also elevated at 6.4 mg/L. A temporal artery biopsy revealed multinucleated giant cells (see Fig. 7.2) and inflammatory infiltrates consistent with giant cell arteritis (GCA).

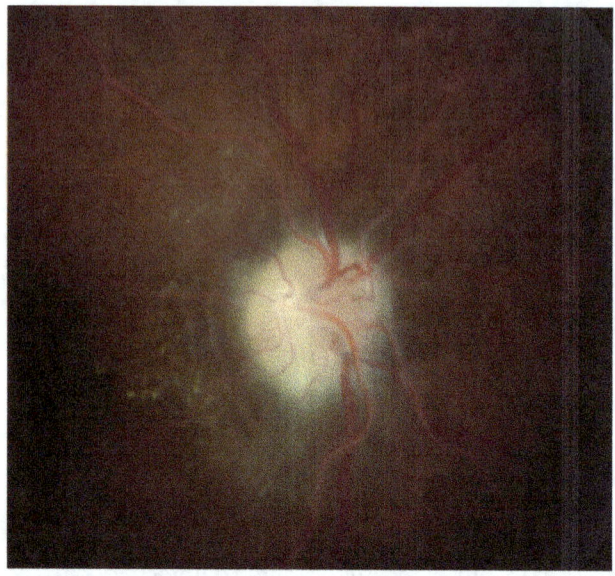

Fig. 7.1. Fundus photograph of the right eye demonstrating optic disc pallor and edema (i.e., pallid edema), a distinctive sign of GCA.

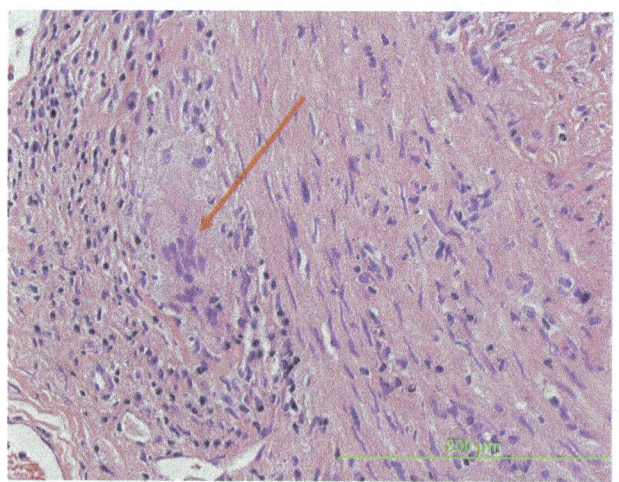

Fig. 7.2. Pathologic specimen from a temporal artery biopsy showing multi-nucleated giant cells (arrow), a distinctive sign of granulomatous inflammation seen in a biopsy specimen positive for GCA.

Question 1	Question 2
Which of the following clinical scenarios is most compatible with arteritic anterior ischemic optic neuropathy (giant cell arteritis)?	Which of the following signs is most suggestive of acute A-AION due to giant cell arteritis (GCA)?
A. 80-year-old woman with slowly progressive, bilateral, painless vision loss for six months **B.** 20-year-old woman with acute, unilateral, painful vision loss **C.** 75-year-old woman with acute, unilateral, painful vision loss **D.** 30-year-old man with acute progressive, bilateral, central painless vision loss	**A.** Pallid optic disc edema **B.** Normal appearing optic nerve **C.** Optociliary shunt vessel **D.** Sectoral optic atrophy
Question 3	Question 4
Which of the following would be the next most appropriate step in a patient in whom GCA is suspected?	Which of the following is the best empiric formula for determining a normal ESR level in men?
A. Temporal artery biopsy **B.** Stat CT without contrast **C.** CBC with differential **D.** Serum ESR and CRP	**A.** Age divided by 10 **B.** (Age − 10)/2 **C.** Age divided by 2 **D.** (Age +10)/2
Question 5	Question 6
Which of the following histopatho-logic findings is most suggestive of GCA?	Which of the following is the recommended timing for performing a temporal artery biopsy after starting steroid treatment?
A. Intact internal elastic lamina **B.** Transmural lymphocytic infiltrate **C.** Multinucleated eosinophils **D.** Non-caseating granulomas	**A.** Must be done within 2 hours **B.** Must be done within 2 days **C.** Less than 2 weeks **D.** Anytime <2 months

Question 7	Question 8
Which of the following immunohisto-chemical stains of epithelioid histiocytes might be useful in adjunctive testing in an initially equivocal temporal artery biopsy?	Which of the following is the best treatment for a patient with suspected GCA with visual loss from A-AION?
A. CD-16 **B.** CD-68 **C.** CD-4 **D.** CD-20	**A.** Oral prednisone 40 mg **B.** Decadron 4 mg immediately **C.** Medrol dose pack **D.** Intravenous methylprednisolone

EXPLANATIONS

The solution to Question 1 is C.

Arteritic anterior ischemic optic neuropathy (A-AION), due to giant cell arteritis (GCA), is a systemic vasculitis that occurs in patients older than 50 years of age, with a mean age of onset of 70 years. GCA is three times more common in women than men, but can occur in either gender. Typical symptoms of GCA include headache, jaw claudication, scalp tenderness, fevers, anorexia, and temporal pain. The most common symptoms are headache or scalp tenderness (occurring in up to 90% of cases), but jaw claudication is highly specific to the diagnosis of GCA. The most common ophthalmologic presentation of GCA is sudden, unilateral vision loss in an elderly patient with variable constitutional symptoms. Up to 40% of patients, however, do not present with classic features (occult GCA) so the clinician must have a high level of suspicion to ask the appropriate questions in these subacute cases.[1-4]

Slowly progressive, painless, bilateral vision loss in an elderly patient would more commonly result from chronic conditions that usually affect both eyes, such as cataracts or macular degeneration. If the chronic central visual loss was due to an optic neuropathy, a compressive or toxic-nutritional etiology would be more likely than GCA to be the etiology. In contrast, a young patient with eye pain (especially with eye movement) and acute vision loss would be more consistent with optic neuritis. A young patient with chronic, progressive, painless, bilateral central vision loss would be most likely to have a chronic toxic, nutritional, or inherited genetic degenerative disease of the retina or optic nerve (e.g., Leber hereditary optic neuropathy in a young man).

The solution to Question 2 is A.

Visual loss in GCA is related to inflammatory-mediated ischemia in the posterior ciliary artery circulation to the optic nerve. In A-AION there may be ischemic infarction as well as disc edema (termed pallid disc edema) which in the acute setting is a differentiating and distinctive sign of GCA (unlike the sectoral or diffuse hyperemic and edematous optic nerve in non-arteritic AION (NAION)). The acute and pallid disc edema of A-AION has been described as a chalky, white-colored optic disc with concomitant edema (see Fig. 7.1). GCA is a systemic vasculitis and thus, in contrast to NAION, can affect more than one ocular vascular supply (retinal, choroidal, or optic nerve). The presence of cotton-wool patches, a non-embolic central retinal artery or cilioretinal artery occlusion, or choroidal hypoperfusion, especially in the setting of AION, should be considered GCA until proven otherwise. As sectoral or diffuse optic atrophy may occur later in the course of both NAION and A-AION, this finding does not differentiate the two entities. A normal disc appearance is more commonly seen in optic neuritis in younger patients (retrobulbar optic neuritis) and would not be typical in AION from either GCA or NAION. The retrobulbar form of ischemic optic neuropathy is termed posterior ischemic optic neuropathy (PION). PION should also be considered to be due to GCA until proven otherwise, as non-arteritic PION is rare (except after general surgical, spine, or cardiac surgeries). Optociliary shunt vessels would be more typically associated with an optic nerve sheath meningioma rather than GCA.

The solution to Question 3 is D.

If the clinical suspicion is high for GCA, then the first test that needs to be performed immediately (we recommend ordering stat for a faster result) is a serum ESR and CRP level. An ESR of at least 40 mm/hr has been included in multiple diagnostic criteria for GCA in the literature, and the American College of Rheumatology classification criteria for GCA includes an ESR of greater than 50 mm/hr. CRP is reported to be more sensitive than ESR and less affected by other extrinsic factors. In one series of over 350 patients, C-reactive protein levels greater than 2.45 mg/dl were reported to be 100% sensitive. The combination of ESR and CRP is more sensitive and specific than either test alone and should be obtained immediately if any clinical suspicion is present. If clinical suspicion is high, steroid treatment should be started immediately, often even before the ESR and CRP results are known. Although a high ESR and/or CRP suggest GCA, in several series, with a positive diagnosis of GCA, the ESR has been reported to be less than 40 mm/hr. Thus, a negative ESR and CRP do not exclude the diagnosis of GCA. In a patient with a high clinical suspicion for GCA, even a borderline ESR or CRP should be suggestive.[2,6–8]

Although a CBC with differential is commonly helpful in the diagnosis of infection, it would not be the first test of choice in GCA. Patients with GCA may have an underlying anemia, however, and the ESR can be affected by marked anemia. An elevated platelet count can also be a marker of an acute inflammatory process in GCA and can assist in the diagnosis, but should not be used as a replacement for ESR and CRP in GCA. CT of the orbits would not be helpful in GCA and would be ordered instead in cases of acute facial trauma, or to diagnose thyroid eye disease. MRI of the brain would be helpful in the setting of acute ischemic stroke but would not be the test of choice in GCA. However, we do recommend neuroimaging for patients with PION to exclude other retrobulbar causes for an optic neuropathy until the diagnosis of GCA is secure. Temporal artery biopsy is the gold standard diagnostic test for GCA, but it can take valuable time to arrange and perform the procedure and to receive the pathologic report; thus, clinical judgment and an ESR/CRP should guide the decision for initial empiric treatment of suspected GCA.

The solution to Question 4 is C.

The ESR (most commonly, the Westergren ESR) is the rate at which red blood cells (RBCs) sediment in a period of one hour (mm/hr). When an inflammatory process is present, increased fibrinogen causes RBC aggregation, which leads to a faster sedimentation rate of RBCs. This process of aggregation, when secondary to an inflammatory process, is referred to as rouleaux formation. Thus, the ESR can be affected by any inflammatory, infectious, or malignant process, or acute stressor that increases the RBC aggregate formation. Therefore, although the ESR is considered a non-specific inflammatory marker which can point to many different disease processes, in the appropriate clinical setting (e.g., elderly patient with headache and visual loss), it is suggestive of GCA. The ESR can also be affected by age and gender, and thus one widely used empiric formula for a normal ESR value is (Age + 10) divided by 2 (used for women) and simply the patient's age divided by 2 (used for men).[9–11] The CRP does not require an age or gender correction for normal values, but we recommend the normal CRP (and not the high sensitivity CRP) for evaluation of GCA.

The solution to Question 5 is B.

GCA is an inflammatory disease involving the recruitment of T-lymphocytes and macrophages which infiltrate large- and medium-sized arteries. The classic histopathological finding on hematoxylin and eosin staining of artery biopsy specimens is granulomatous inflammation. Caseating granulomas are not found in GCA, and are instead more consistent with a diagnosis of a granulomatous infection, such as tuberculosis. Non-caseating granulomas are the hallmark of sarcoidosis. Lymphocytes, macrophages, and multinucleated giant cells are most commonly located at the intima-media junction, although the inflammatory infiltrate can also extend through all layers of the arterial wall (transmural inflammation). There is often disruption of the elastic lamina. However, these findings are only present in approximately 50% of cases, and up to one third of temporal artery biopsy results may be normal. In a series of 28 cases where arteritis was suspected but temporal artery biopsy was negative, GCA was still considered the diagnosis in 12 of the 28 patients. Thus, even with a negative biopsy, if the clinical suspicion for GCA is high, the diagnosis of GCA cannot be excluded.[1–3,12]

The solution to Question 6 is C.

In cases of suspected GCA, a biopsy should be performed as soon as possible, but it is generally considered reasonable to perform a temporal artery biopsy within 14 days of diagnosis, even after initial steroid treatment. Although some studies report a higher biopsy yield before 14 days and increased atypical features and deviation from the normal histopathologic findings after 14 days of treatment, a temporal artery biopsy does not have to be performed within hours to days of diagnosis to be positive for GCA. If a biopsy cannot be performed within 14 days, there can still be pathological value in performing a biopsy, but a negative result must be taken with the consideration that it could be a false negative. Even so, some studies have demonstrated positive biopsies revealing GCA up to 45 days after steroid treatment.[1,13–15]

The solution to Question 7 is B.

CD-68 is a glycoprotein expressed on cells with a monocyte/macrophage lineage. CD-68 has been demonstrated to be a useful adjunctive immunohistochemical marker in the diagnosis of GCA on temporal artery biopsy. If no macrophages can be definitively identified visually using conventional hematoxylin and eosin staining, CD-68 can be used to stain macrophages to better highlight their presence or absence in the specimen. CD-16 can be found in some populations of monocytes but has not been demonstrated to be useful in the diagnosis of GCA.[16–17] We use CD-68 and the Movat pentachrome (specific for the internal elastic lamina) in cases of equivocal histologic evaluations for GCA in a temporal artery biopsy. The presence of focal disruption of the internal elastic lamina on the Movat pentachrome, adjacent fibrosis, and positive CD-68 staining can help to make the diagnosis of healed temporal arteritis in these cases. CD-4 and CD-20 are both used to identify T- and B-lymphocytes which would indicate an inflammatory process, but would not be helpful in differentiating GCA from other types of inflammation.

The solution to Question 8 is D.

Corticosteroids are the established initial treatment of choice for GCA and should be administered as soon as possible when the diagnosis is suspected (even before temporal artery biopsy confirmation). Early administration of steroids has been demonstrated to reduce the incidence and severity of blindness and can rapidly improve the patient's clinical symptoms. Initial treatment requires high doses beginning with 60–100 mg per day of oral prednisone (1–1.5 mg/kg dose). Although some rheumatologic literature suggests lower doses of oral prednisone (40 mg) might be effective in GCA, we do not recommend this lower dose for patients with visual loss and GCA. If visual symptoms are present, high doses of 1–1.5 mg/kg/day of oral prednisone or IV steroids are recommended. We do not believe that there is any role for the Medrol dose pack in GCA. Although there has been no head-to-head, randomized controlled clinical trial comparing IV to oral steroids in GCA, we generally recommend IV methylprednisolone for GCA patients with visual loss.

If the patient cannot tolerate prednisone, is having severe steroid-related side effects, or requires chronic treatment and cannot come off steroids, secondary immunosuppressant treatment (e.g., methotrexate) may be added under the supervision of rheumatology. Long-term steroid treatment is notorious for significant side effects and although new treatment regimens and agents are currently under investigation, steroids are still considered the first-line, immediate treatment for GCA.[1–3,18,19]

SUMMARY

Arteritic anterior ischemic optic neuropathy (A-AION) due to GCA is a common systemic vasculitis of the elderly that affects the medium- and large-sized arteries. It most commonly presents in patients above the age of 50 years with acute vision loss that may be unilateral or bilateral. GCA is often associated with general symptoms including headache, jaw claudication, temporal pain, scalp tenderness, fever, and anorexia. The classic ophthalmoscopic exam finding is pallid edema, but AION accompanied by ischemia in another vascular supply (such as the central retinal artery or choroidal vasculature) should suggest GCA. Likewise, PION in an elderly patient should suggest GCA over retrobulbar optic neuritis. An ESR and CRP must be performed as soon as possible (preferably stat). However, if clinical suspicion is high for GCA, then high-dose oral or IV steroids should be initiated as soon as possible and treatment should not be delayed waiting for laboratory or biopsy results. Although the gold standard for diagnosis is a temporal artery biopsy, it can be performed safely within two weeks of starting treatment. The TA biopsy has a relatively high sensitivity (96%) and a high specificity. If, however, the biopsy is negative and the clinical suspicion for GCA remains high, then the other side should be strongly considered for biopsy to confirm diagnosis, as GCA can have pathologic areas of skip lesions (regions of the artery that are not inflamed separated by inflamed regions). The classic histological findings for GCA include intimal thickening, transmural inflammation, infiltration of lymphocytes, CD-68+ macrophages, and multinucleated giant cells, as well as destruction of the internal elastic lamina. Steroids are typically required for months to several years, but adjunctive immunosuppression may be necessary in some patients. Serial ESR and CRP tests, in conjunction with clinical findings, are used to help taper the steroids. Once vision loss has occurred, steroids are unlikely to restore vision, but immediate diagnosis and steroid treatment are crucial to prevent involvement of the fellow eye.

REFERENCES

1. Waldman CW, Waldman SD, Waldman RA. (2013) Giant cell arteritis. *Med Clin North Am* **98**:329–335.
2. Salvarani C, Cantinia F, Hunder GG. (2008) Polymalgia rheumatica and giant-cell arteritis. *Lancet* **372**:234–245.
3. Levine SM, Hellmann DB. (2002) Giant cell arteritis. *Curr Opin Rheumatol* **14**:3–10.
4. Hayreh SS. (2009) Ischemic optic neuropathy. *Prog Retin Eye Res* **28**:34–62.

5. Kerr NM, Chew S, Danesh-Meyer HV. (2009) Non-arteritic anterior ischaemic optic neuropathy: a review and update. *J Clin Neurosci* **16**:994–1000.

6. Hunder GG, Bloch DA, Michel BA, *et al*. (1990) The American College of Rheumatology 1990 criteria for the classification of giant cell arteritis. *Arthritis Rheum* **33**:1122–1128.

7. Salvarani C, Hunder GG. (2001) Giant cell arteritis with low erythrocyte sedimentation rate: frequency of occurrence in a population-based study. *Arthritis Rheum* **45**:140–145.

8. Hayreh SS, Podhajsky PA, Raman R, Zimmerman B. (1997) Giant cell arteritis: validity and reliability of various diagnostic criteria. *Am J Ophthalmol* **123**: 285–296.

9. Miller A, Green M, Robinson D. (1983) Simple rule for calculating normal erythrocyte sedimentation rate. *Br Med J (Clin Res Ed)* **286**:266.

10. Fabry TL. (1987) Mechanism of erythrocyte aggregation and sedimentation. *Blood* **70**:1572–1576.

11. American Association for Clinical Chemistry. (2010) *ESR: The Test*. Available at: http://labtestsonline.org/understanding/analytes/esr/tab/test [Accessed Aug 2013].

12. Esteban MJ, Font C, Hernandez-Rodriguez J, *et al*. (2001) Small-vessel vasculitis surrounding a spared temporal artery: clinical and pathological findings in a series of twenty-eight patients. *Arthritis Rheum* **44**:1387–1395.

13. Ray-Chaudhuri N, Kine DA, Tijani SO, *et al*. (2002) Effect of prior steroid treatment on temporal artery biopsy findings in giant cell arteritis. *Br J Ophthalmol* **86**:530–532.

14. Narvaez J, Bernad B, Roig-Vilaseca D, *et al*. (2007) Influence of previous corticosteroid therapy on temporal artery biopsy yield in giant cell arteritis. *Semin Arthritis Rheum* **37**:13–19.

15. Achkar AA, Lie JT, Hunder GG, *et al*. (1994) How does previous corticosteroid treatment affect the biopsy findings in giant cell (temporal) arteritis? *Ann Intern Med* **120**:987–992.

16. Font RL, Prabhakaran VC. (2007) Histological parameters helpful in recognising steroid-treated temporal arteritis: an analysis of 35 cases. *Br J Ophthalmol* **91**:204–209.

17. The Immunology Link. (2010) *Human CD Antigens CD1 to CD100*. Available at: http://www.immunologylink.com/cdantigen1.html [Accessed Aug 2013].

18. Hayreh SS, Zimmerman B, Kardon RH. (2002) Visual improvement with corticosteroid therapy in giant cell arteritis. Report of a large study and review of literature. *Acta Ophthalmol Scand* **80**:355–367.

19. Salvarani C, Cantini F, Boiardi L, Hunder GG. (2002) Polymyalgia rheumatica and giant-cell arteritis. *N Engl J Med* **347**:261–271.

8

Thyroid Eye Disease

Arielle Spitze MD, Alexander S. Davis MD,
Nagham Al-Zubidi MD, Sushma Yalamanchili MD,
and Andrew G. Lee MD

CASE

A 53-year-old woman presented with subacute, progressive, painless, bilateral vision loss over the previous six months. Past medical history was significant for hypertension, hyperlipidemia, and Graves disease that was well controlled on propylthiouracil (PTU). She was an active smoker of one pack per day (PPD) of cigarettes with a total 35-pack-year history. Best-corrected vision was 20/300 in the right eye (OD) and 20/400 in the left eye (OS). External exam demonstrated bilateral proptosis (Fig. 8.1), with Hertel exophthalmometer measurements of 27 mm in both eyes (OU). Pupils were 5 mm in the dark and 3 mm in the light OU, with no relative afferent pupillary defect (RAPD). Extraocular movements demonstrated a bilateral, right greater than left global ophthalmoplegia. Intraocular pressures were elevated bilaterally at 28 mmHg OD and 25 mmHg OS. Automated visual fields (Humphrey 24-2) demonstrated bilateral central/cecocentral scotomas (Fig. 8.2). External examination demonstrated periorbital erythema and edema, as well as upper and lower lid retraction. Slit lamp biomicroscopy showed moderate conjunctival injection, and inferior corneal punctate epithelial erosions OU. Dilated fundus exam demonstrated a cup-to-disc ratio of 0.2 with bilateral temporal optic nerve atrophy (Fig. 8.3). Magnetic resonance imaging (MRI) of the brain and orbit without contrast was performed

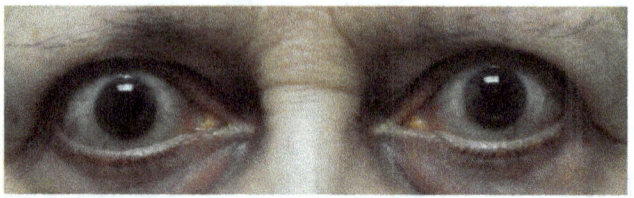

Fig. 8.1. External photo of patient with evidence of bilateral lid retraction, inferior scleral show, and proptosis.

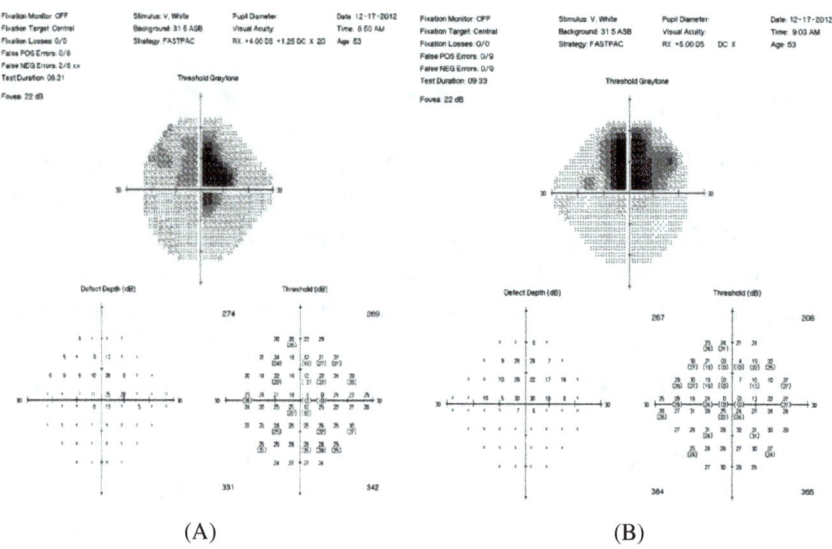

(A)   (B)

Fig. 8.2. Visual field demonstrating cecocentral scotomas bilaterally. (A) Visual field of the left eye. (B) Visual field of the right eye.

at an outside institution just prior to evaluation, which demonstrated proptosis and enlarged extraocular muscles with sparing of the tendinous sheaths OU and compression of the optic nerve at the orbital apex bilaterally (Fig. 8.4).

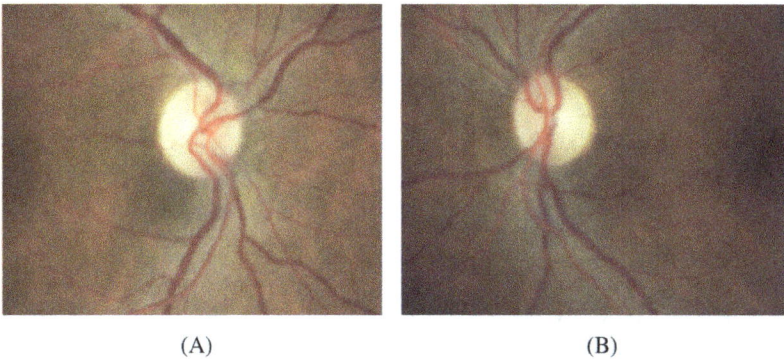

(A)   (B)

Fig. 8.3. Fundus photos demonstrating bilateral temporal pallor. (A) Fundus photo of the right eye. (B) Fundus photo of the left eye.

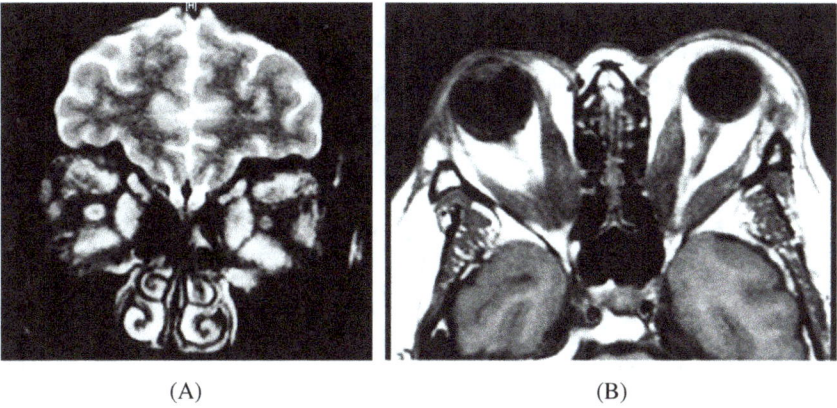

(A)   (B)

Fig. 8.4. MRI of the orbit without contrast. (A) T2 coronal view demonstrating significantly enlarged extraocular muscles. (B) Axial view demonstrating muscle enlargement with tendon sparing.

Question 1	Question 2
Which of the following is the most likely presenting symptom of thyroid eye disease (TED)?	**Which of the following is the most likely sign in TED?**
A. Intermittent binocular diplopia **B.** Transient altitudinal visual field loss **C.** Variable and fatigable ptosis **D.** Episodic pupillary mydriasis	**A.** Eyelid retraction **B.** Eyelid ptosis **C.** Superior oblique weakness **D.** Incomitant exotropia
Question 3	Question 4
Which of the following tests would be most suggestive of TED in a patient with known hypothyroidism?	**Which of the following is the best initial imaging study for TED in a patient with poorly controlled hyperthyroidism?**
A. Thyroid-stimulating hormone **B.** TSIg and TPO antibodies **C.** Serum T4 and T3 levels **D.** Thyroid ultrasound for goiter	**A.** MRI of the head with/without contrast **B.** Computed tomography (CT) of the head without contrast **C.** CT of the orbits without contrast **D.** CT of the orbits with contrast
Question 5	Question 6
Which of the following clinical signs is most consistent with a compressive optic neuropathy in TED?	**Which of the following is the best initial step in a patient with confirmed TED?**
A. Global ophthalmoplegia **B.** Marked anisocoria **C.** Severe proptosis **D.** Small RAPD	**A.** Control of thyroid levels **B.** Orbital decompression surgery **C.** Oral prednisone at a weight-adjusted dose **D.** Orbital low-dose irradiation

EXPLANATIONS

The solution to Question 1 is A.

Thyroid eye disease (TED), also known as thyroid or Graves ophthalmopathy, thyroid orbitopathy, or thyroid-associated ophthalmopathy, is the ocular manifestation of autoimmune thyroid disease and represents the most common disease affecting the orbit in adults. TED affects approximately 40–60% of patients with Graves disease,[1–3] with a female predilection[4] of 3.45:1 (female:male).[5] Dry eyes, blurred vision, and monocular and binocular diplopia are all commonly described symptoms of TED. Dry eye symptoms in patients with TED are very common and can produce monocular diplopia. Blurred vision can be due to underlying refractive error (e.g., induced hyperopic or astigmatic error) or abnormalities/deficiencies in the tear film,[6] but clinicians should perform additional testing to exclude a compressive optic neuropathy in TED. Intermittent binocular diplopia is a common symptom, as many patients have intermittent fusional control of their deviation in primary gaze. Other patients may only complain of diplopia in extremes of gaze. Patients with dry eye from TED can experience transient monocular or bilateral visual blurring, but transient altitudinal visual field loss (amaurosis fugax) is a more typical sign of transient ischemia than TED. Variable ptosis, especially with fatigue, is the hallmark of myasthenia gravis (MG). MG can however, occur concomitantly with TED. Episodic mydriasis is a finding in benign episodic pupillary dilation and is not related to TED.

The solution to Question 2 is A.

One of the most distinct and often earliest signs of TED is eyelid retraction, occurring in some studies in greater than 90% of patients[3,7,8] (see Fig. 8.1, demonstrating bilateral upper and lower lid retraction and proptosis). The absence of lid retraction in TED should prompt a more thorough workup to explore other etiologies. Other clinical signs typically seen with TED can include chemosis, conjunctival hyperemia, periorbital edema or injection, inferior scleral show,[9,10] and superior limbic keratoconjunctivitis.[11,12] Myasthenia gravis is also autoimmune-mediated, explaining its higher rate of co-occurrence in patients diagnosed with autoimmune thyroid disease.[13] Myasthenia gravis should be considered whenever a patient presents with fatigable ptosis, variable cranial nerve palsies, or ptosis co-existing with TED. TED typically does not cause ptosis of the eyelids, but rather, retraction and lid lag on downward gaze. However, if lid retraction is asymmetric, this can be mistaken for ptosis in the unaffected eye as compared to the affected eye with lid retraction. Restrictive extraocular motility or myopathy is common in patients with TED. The typical percentage of muscle involvement is as follows: inferior and medial rectus (in 75% of cases), and superior and lateral rectus (less commonly, in 50% of cases).[14] The order of extraocular muscle enlargement is (1) inferior recti (43%); (2) medial recti (38%); (3) superior recti (29%); (4) lateral recti (16%)[15] (see extraocular muscle enlargement demonstrated in the MRI in Fig. 8.4). Thus, the typical deviation in thyroid eye disease is esotropia from a tight medial rectus muscle and hypotropia from a tight inferior rectus muscle and not exotropia from lateral rectus involvement, which is the least likely muscle to be involved in TED. A careful pupil examination is required in TED because a RAPD can be present if the patient has unilateral or bilateral but asymmetric damage to either of the optic nerves from compressive optic neuropathy.[16,17] However, bilateral involvement of TED can commonly[18] occur[19]; thus, if there are bilateral, approximately equal optic neuropathies, no RAPD would be expected due to a lack of relative difference between the afferent pathways of each optic nerve. Sometimes, a bilateral defect in the afferent pupillary pathway can be confirmed by light-near dissociation OU.

The solution to Question 3 is B.

The diagnosis and evaluation of TED first involves laboratory testing with a thyroid function panel, including thyroid-stimulating hormone (TSH), T3, T4, and consideration for thyroid auto-antibodies (e.g., anti-thyroid peroxidase antibody (TPO) and thyroid-stimulating immunoglobulin (TSIg)).[20] It is of note that although TED is commonly described in the literature as being associated with hyperthyroidism (Graves disease), patients may have TED with hypothyroid (especially after treated hyperthyroidism)[4] or euthyroid states (treated or untreated).[21] In addition, other non-autoimmune etiologies can produce systemic thyroid disease (e.g., surgical thyroidectomy for thyroid cancer). Thus, neither the presence nor absence of systemic hyperthyroidism by laboratory testing should exclude the clinical diagnosis of TED. Thyroid ultrasound may be helpful in evaluating the systemic disease but orbital ultrasound is more diagnostic for TED (e.g., extraocular muscle enlargement). The presence of thyroid auto-antibodies (TSIg and anti-TPO) in a patient with known hypothyroidism and clinical and/or radiographic findings of TED is highly supportive of the diagnosis.

The solution to Question 4 is C.

The most commonly used initial imaging study in the evaluation of a patient with suspected TED is a CT of the orbits without contrast.[18] Imaging is useful for confirming the clinical diagnosis (enlarged extraocular muscles); for establishing the relationship of the enlarged muscles to the optic nerve in cases of optic neuropathy; and for assisting in the preparation for surgical decompression if surgical treatment is required at any time in the future.[15] The contrast material used for CT scans is iodinated and should probably be avoided in any patient with suspected active Graves disease, as it may cause or worsen systemic thyrotoxicosis in rare patients. Furthermore, contrast is not necessary to demonstrate the distinctive radiographic finding of enlarged extraocular muscles in TED.[22] MRI imaging, however, may have advantages demonstrating radiographic evidence of optic nerve compression or active edema on T2-weighted imaging, but in general, CT of the orbit is sufficient for imaging TED. MRI may have some advantages for radiographic evidence of optic nerve compression or for demonstrating active edema on T2-weighted imaging but in general CT of the orbit is sufficient for TED.[23] MRI of the orbit and head with contrast and fat suppression might be useful however for cases where TED is not the only consideration in the differential diagnosis; MRI can also be helpful to distinguish intracranial lesions with intraorbital extension (e.g., orbitocranial meningioma), which can mimic the clinical presentation of TED. Standardized A-scan ultrasonography can also be performed to measure extraocular muscle size to confirm muscle enlargement in patients with TED,[24] but is very institution and operator dependent and not universally available. Thus we generally recommend an orbital CT (or less commonly an MRI) as the first-line evaluation of suspected compressive optic neuropathy in TED.[14,18]

The solution to Question 5 is D.

A decrease in visual acuity can occur in a patient with TED secondary to refractive changes or due to tear film abnormalities,[6] but this must be differentiated from decreased visual acuity secondary to an optic neuropathy, where a RAPD would be detected on the affected side (assuming the optic neuropathy is not equal in both eyes). Compressive optic neuropathy can cause a subtle and progressive loss of visual acuity and requires a full examination including testing of automated visual fields (see Fig. 8.2), color testing for dyschromatopsia, and evaluation of the pupils for the presence of a RAPD. Although exophthalmometry is important in TED, the presence of proptosis does not necessarily correlate with an optic neuropathy.[25] In fact, the presence of proptosis may act as a natural "decompression" by displacing orbital tissues anteriorly,[18] effectively protecting against optic nerve compression in many cases. Similarly, while the extraocular motility examination can often be abnormal or reveal extraocular muscle restriction in TED, this alone does not imply that an optic neuropathy is present. Marked global ophthalmoplegia might, however, suggest a crowded orbit, which could predispose the formation of a TED-related compressive optic neuropathy. Some additional concerning signs that may indicate more urgent consideration for surgical intervention in TED: (1) elevated intraocular pressure measurements, particularly in upgaze,[26–28] which can be measured with portable tonometry (i.e., Tono-Pen); (2) optic disc edema or pallor on fundus examination (but compressive optic neuropathy can have a normal-appearing optic nerve)[29]; or (3) severe or progressive visual loss. Although any visual field defect may occur, the most common visual field defects observed in TED-related compressive optic neuropathies include paracentral or cecocentral scotomas (see Fig. 8.2), inferior altitudinal defects, and enlarged blind spots.[29]

The solution to Question 6 is A.

The best initial workup of all patients with TED is prompt evaluation and management by primary care or endocrinology to ensure a stable and euthyroid state, as dysthyroid states (both hyperthyroidism and hypothyroidism) have been associated with more severe TED.[30] Another important discussion during the initial visit of every TED patient is cigarette smoking, since cessation of smoking has been shown to significantly reduce progression and even decrease the occurrence of TED.[31–34]

Depending on the severity of TED, medical, surgical, or a combination of interventions can be used for treatment based on each patient's symptoms and signs. Aggressive lubrication with artificial tears and ointment is helpful to prevent exposure keratopathy. The concurrent use of steroids (oral or IV, depending on severity), or low-dose orbital radiation in the acute phase of TED can decrease orbital inflammation or congestion. The natural course of TED as described by Rundle's curve is an initial acute phase, which then peaks and then leads to a chronic, stable phase.[35] Treatment decisions will differ depending on where the disease falls on Rundle's curve. If there is evidence of compressive optic neuropathy in TED, then urgent imaging and consideration for orbital decompression should be made. Following orbital and/or fat decompression, further surgical treatment may be needed, including strabismus or lid surgery. In general, the surgical procedures for TED should be performed in this order, as orbital surgery can affect the eye position within the orbit and strabismus surgery can affect the lid position.[6,35] However, some patients who do not require either orbit or strabismus surgery may benefit from lid surgery only for reconstructive and cosmetic purposes.

SUMMARY

Thyroid eye disease is an autoimmune-mediated disorder producing orbital fat and muscle inflammation in patients with dysthyroid (but sometimes euthyroid) states. Cross-reactivity of orbital and thyroid antigens with secondary inflammation is believed to be the cause of TED. TED affects females more than males (3.45:1), more commonly occurs after the age of 40 years, and typically occurs at or following the onset of the dysthyroid state.[36] The most commonly encountered symptoms and signs include decreased vision, dry eye symptoms, diplopia, lid retraction, proptosis, dysmotility, chemosis, conjunctival hyperemia, superior limbic keratoconjunctivitis, and inferior scleral show. In severe cases, compressive optic neuropathy may occur (decreased visual acuity, visual field defects, RAPD, color vision abnormalities), which can also be associated with increased intraocular pressure measurements, disc edema, or pallor. Myasthenia gravis should be considered whenever a patient presents with new or fatigable ptosis, variable cranial nerve palsies, and can co-exist with TED. Patients with severe disease (e.g., compressive optic neuropathy) generally require orbital imaging confirmation of TED and should be evaluated preferably with CT of the orbits without contrast in the acute, hyperthyroid state. MRI of the orbits can show additional findings in TED but in general is more expensive than orbital CT. Ultrasound is less expensive than CT or MR scanning but is operator dependent and not universally available. Stabilization of systemic thyroid levels to maintain a euthyroid state and smoking cessation if applicable are the first steps. Aggressive lubrication may be helpful if exposure keratopathy is present. In the acute phase, oral or IV pulse steroids may be helpful in TED. Low-dose orbital radiation is controversial but might be useful for reducing active orbital inflammation. For patients with severe TED requiring surgical therapy, orbital decompression, followed by strabismus surgery, and finally lid surgery, can be performed, and generally should follow this order. Compressive optic neuropathy is the most feared complication of TED and patients who fail maximum medical therapy or present with acute or progressive severe visual loss should be treated aggressively, including consideration for urgent orbital decompression.

REFERENCES

1. Wiersinga WM, Bartalena L. (2002) Epidemiology and prevention of Graves' ophthalmopathy. *Thyroid* **12**:855–860.
2. Soeters MR, van Zeijl CJ, Boelen A, *et al.* (2011) Optimal management of Graves orbitopathy: a multidisciplinary approach. *Neth J Med* **69**:302–308.

3. Maheshwari R, Weis E. (2012) Thyroid associated orbitopathy. *Indian J Ophthalmol* **60**:87–93.
4. Lazarus JH. (2012) Epidemiology of Graves' orbitopathy (GO) and relationship with thyroid disease. *Best Pract Res Clin Endocrinol Metab* **26**:273–279.
5. Gupta A, Sadeghi PB, Akpek EK. (2009) Occult thyroid eye disease in patients presenting with dry eye symptoms. *Am J Ophthalmol* **147**:919–923.
6. Perros P, Neoh C, Dickinson J. (2009) Thyroid eye disease. *BMJ* **338**:b560.
7. Cruz AA, Ribeiro SF, Garcia DM, *et al.* (2013) Graves upper eyelid retraction. *Surv Ophthalmol* **58**:63–76.
8. Gould DJ, Roth FS, Soparkar CN. (2012) The diagnosis and treatment of thyroid-associated ophthalmopathy. *Aesthetic Plast Surg* **36**:638–648.
9. Feldman KA, Putterman AM, Farber MD. (1992) Surgical treatment of thyroid-related lower eyelid retraction: a modified approach. *Ophthal Plast Reconstr Surg* **8**:278–286.
10. Thaller VT, Kaden K, Lane CM, Collin JR. (1987) Thyroid lid surgery. *Eye (Lond)* **1**:609–614.
11. Kadrmas EF, Bartley GB. (1995) Superior limbic keratoconjunctivitis. A prognostic sign for severe Graves ophthalmopathy. *Ophthalmology* **102**:1472–1475.
12. Chavis PS. (2002) Thyroid and the eye. *Curr Opin Ophthalmol* **13**:352–356.
13. Chen YL, Yeh JH, Chiu HC. (2012) Clinical features of myasthenia gravis patients with autoimmune thyroid disease in Taiwan. *Acta Neurol Scand* **127**:170–174.
14. Becker M, Masterson K, Delavelle J, *et al.* (2010) Imaging of the optic nerve. *Eur J Radiol* **74**:299–313.
15. Goncalves AC, Gebrim EM, Monteiro ML. (2012) Imaging studies for diagnosing Graves' orbitopathy and dysthyroid optic neuropathy. *Clinics (Sao Paulo)* **67**:1327–1334.
16. Jeon C, Shin JH, Woo KI, Kim YD. (2012) Clinical profile and visual outcomes after treatment in patients with dysthyroid optic neuropathy. *Korean J Ophthalmol* **26**:73–79.
17. Bahn RS, Bartley GB, Gorman CA. (1992) Emergency treatment of Graves' ophthalmopathy. *Baillieres Clin Endocrinol Metab* **6**:95–105.
18. Rose JG Jr, Burkat CN, Boxrud CA. (2005) Diagnosis and management of thyroid orbitopathy. *Otolaryngol Clin North Am* **38**:1043–1074.
19. Enzmann DR, Donaldson SS, Kriss JP. (1979) Appearance of Graves' disease on orbital computed tomography. *J Comput Assist Tomogr* **3**:815–819.
20. Swain M, Swain T, Mohanty BK. (2005) Autoimmune thyroid disorders — an update. *Indian J Clin Biochem* **20**:9–17.
21. Eckstein A, Esser J, Mann K, Schott M. (2010) Clinical value of TSH receptor antibodies measurement in patients with Graves' orbitopathy. *Pediatr Endocrinol Rev 7* **Suppl 2**:198–203.
22. Van der Molen AJ, Thomsen HS, Morcos SK. (2004) Effect of iodinated contrast media on thyroid function in adults. *Eur Radiol* **14**:902–907.

23. Dodds NI, Atcha AW, Birchall D, Jackson A. (2009) Use of high-resolution MRI of the optic nerve in Graves' ophthalmopathy. *Br J Radiol* **82**:541–544.

24. Yamamoto K, Saito K, Takai T, Yoshida S. (1983) Diagnosis of exophthalmos using orbital ultrasonography and treatment of malignant exophthalmos with steroid therapy, orbital radiation therapy, and plasmapheresis. *Prog Clin Biol Res* **116**:189–205.

25. Frueh BR, Musch DC, Garber FW. (1986) Exophthalmometer readings in patients with Graves' eye disease. *Ophthalmic Surg* **17**:37–40.

26. Norris JH, Ross JJ, Kazim M, *et al.* (2012) The effect of orbital decompression surgery on refraction and intraocular pressure in patients with thyroid orbitopathy. *Eye (Lond)* **26**:535–543.

27. Haefliger IO, von Arx G, Pimentel AR. (2010) Pathophysiology of intraocular pressure increase and glaucoma prevalence in thyroid eye disease: a mini-review. *Klin Monbl Augenheilkd* **227**:292–293.

28. Gamblin GT, Galentine P, Chernow B, *et al.* (1985) Evidence of extraocular muscle restriction in autoimmune thyroid disease. *J Clin Endocrinol Metab* **61**:167–171.

29. Neigel JM, Rootman J, Belkin RI, *et al.* (1988) Dysthyroid optic neuropathy. The crowded orbital apex syndrome. *Ophthalmology* **95**:1515–1521.

30. Prummel MF, Wiersinga WM, Mourits MP, *et al.* (1990) Effect of abnormal thyroid function on the severity of Graves' ophthalmopathy. *Arch Intern Med* **150**:1098–1101.

31. Cawood TJ, Moriarty P, O'Farrelly C, O'Shea D. (2007) Smoking and thyroid-associated ophthalmopathy: a novel explanation of the biological link. *J Clin Endocrinol Metab* **92**:59–64.

32. Garrity JA, Bahn RS. (2006) Pathogenesis of graves ophthalmopathy: implications for prediction, prevention, and treatment. *Am J Ophthalmol* **142**:147–153.

33. Bartalena L. (2012) Prevention of Graves' ophthalmopathy. *Best Pract Res Clin Endocrinol Metab* **26**:371–379.

34. Lee JH, Lee SY, Yoon JS. (2010) Risk factors associated with the severity of thyroid-associated orbitopathy in Korean patients. *Korean J Ophthalmol* **24**:267–273.

35. Bothun ED, Scheurer RA, Harrison AR, Lee MS. (2009) Update on thyroid eye disease and management. *Clin Ophthalmol* **3**:543–551.

36. Kendler DL, Lippa J, Rootman J. (1993) The initial clinical characteristics of Graves' orbitopathy vary with age and sex. *Arch Ophthalmol* **111**:197–201.

9

Optic Neuritis

Nagham Al-Zubidi MD, Arielle Spitze MD, Sushma Yalamanchili MD, and Andrew G. Lee MD

CASE

A 35-year-old female presented with a two-week history of worsening vision and pain with eye movement in the left eye (OS). She denied any other neurological symptoms, family history of multiple sclerosis, toxic exposure, recent travel or sick contacts, pets, or any history of sexually transmitted disease. The remainder of her medical history was unremarkable. On examination, her best-corrected visual acuity was 20/20 in the right eye (OD) and 20/400 OS. Pupils were equal and measured 5 mm in the dark and 3 mm in the light and there was a left relative afferent pupillary defect (RAPD). Color vision plates were 14/14 OD and 0/14 OS. Extraocular movements were full in all gaze positions. Intraocular pressure measurements and slit lamp examination were normal in both eyes (OU). Automated visual fields (Humphrey 24-2) revealed diffuse depression of the visual field OS and was normal OD (Fig. 9.1). Dilated funduscopic examination was normal OU (Fig. 9.2). Magnetic resonance imaging (MRI) of the brain and orbits with and without gadolinium and fat suppression demonstrated enhancement of the left optic nerve on T1 post-contrast images. No white matter lesions were detected on T2 fluid-attenuated inversion recovery (FLAIR) sequences (Fig. 9.3).

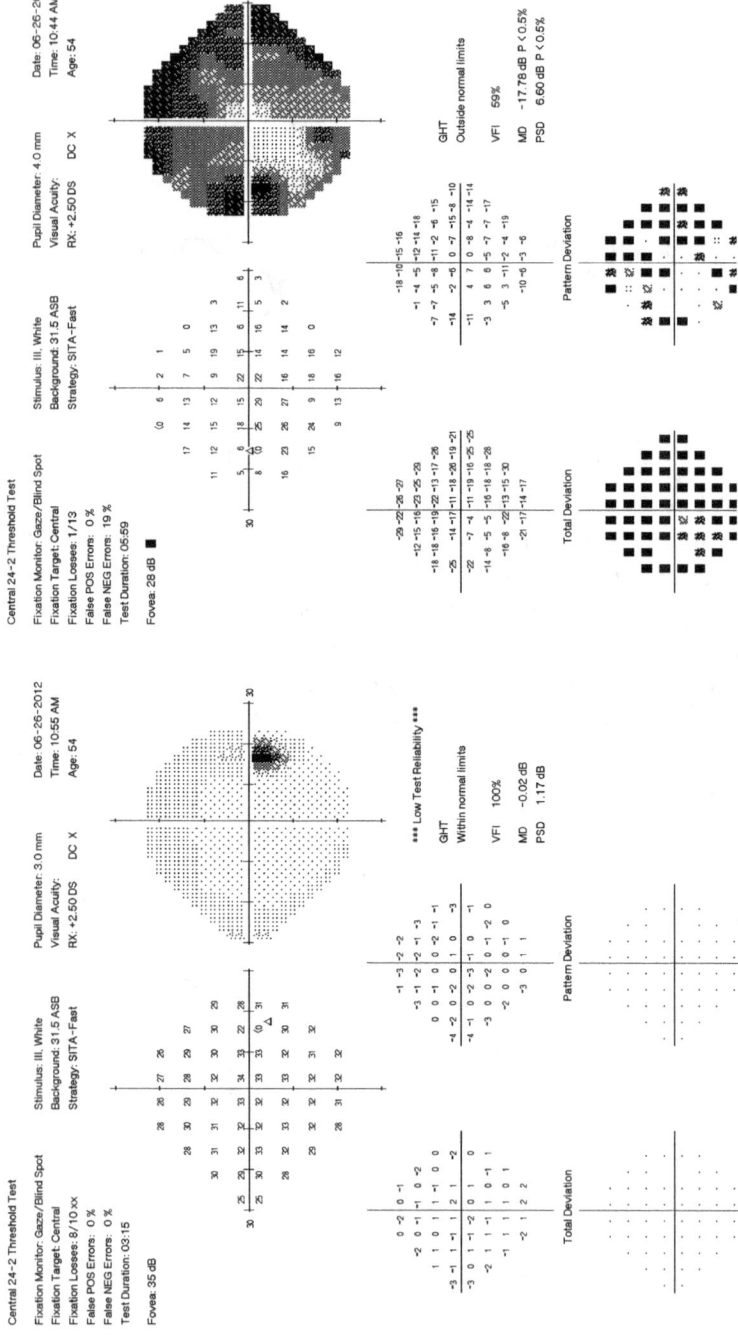

Fig. 9.1. Patient's Humphrey visual fields (24-2) showing diffuse depression visual field defect OS and appearing normal OD.

Question 1	Question 2
Which of the following symptoms is most consistent with demyelinating optic neuritis (ON) in adults?	**Which of the following signs is most consistent with typical demyelinating adult ON?**
A. Unilateral vision loss and pain B. Bilateral painful vision loss C. Unilateral painless vision loss D. Bilateral painless vision loss	A. Marked optic disc edema B. Normal-appearing optic nerves C. Disc edema with a macular star figure D. Optic atrophy in one eye
Question 3	Question 4
A 40-year-old woman had optic neuritis OD but was left with a residual visual field defect and optic atrophy. She now presents with visual loss OS and very poorly reactive pupils OU but no RAPD. Which of the following pupillary test results suggests a bilateral symmetric optic neuropathy?	**Which of the following types of visual field defect is most likely in demyelinating ON?**
A. Constriction to dilute pilocarpine B. Light-near dissociation C. Denervation supersensitivity D. Pupil dilation lag in the dark	A. Bitemporal hemianopsia B. Homonymous hemianopsia C. Junctional scotoma D. Central scotoma
Question 5	Question 6
Which of the following is the best imaging study for an acute unilateral optic neuropathy?	**Which of the following is the best indication for ordering neuromyelitis optica (NMO) antibody in ON?**
A. Diffusion-weighted imaging (DWI) on MRI B. Cranial computed tomography (CT) scan and CT angiography (CTA) C. MRI of the orbit with gadolinium contrast D. Contrast cranial and orbital MRI with fat saturation	A. Retrobulbar optic neuropathy OD B. Optic disc edema with a macular star figure OD C. Bilateral optic neuritis with poor recovery D. Unilateral optic neuritis with recovery of vision

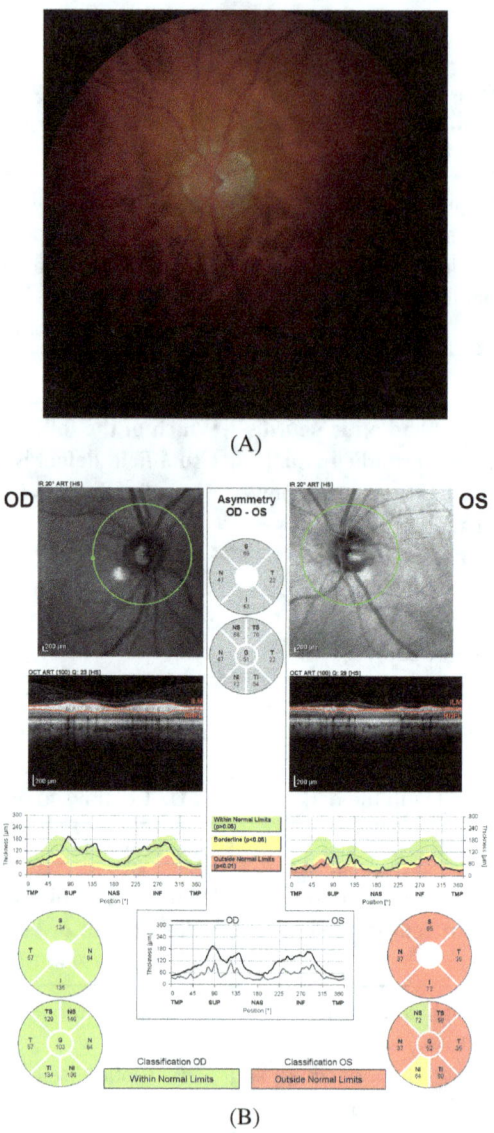

Fig. 9.2. (A) Normal-appearing left optic disc in 35-year-old female with optic neuritis. (B) OCT showing left optic nerve fiber layer loss over time due to optic atrophy OS.

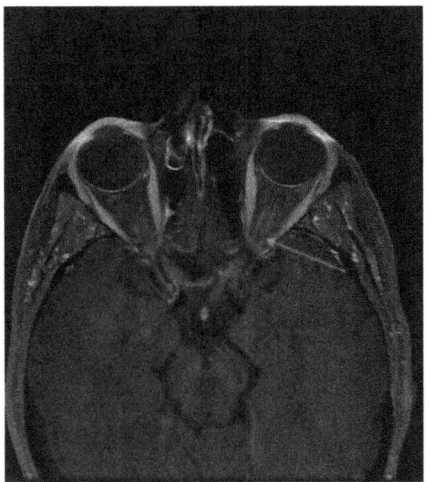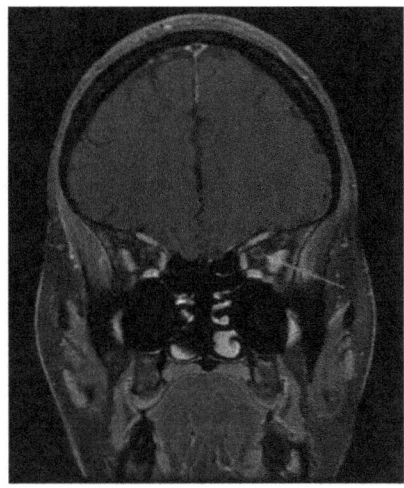

Fig. 9.3. Coronal and axial T1 post-gadolinium, fat-suppressed MRI showing the typical enhancement of the left optic nerve seen in ON.

Question 7	Question 8
According to the Optic Neuritis Treatment Trial (ONTT), which of the following is the best treatment for acute demyelinating optic neuritis?	**According to the ONTT, which of the following is the predicted 15-year risk of developing multiple sclerosis (MS) based upon an initial MRI scan with multiple periventricular white matter lesions?**
A. IV methylprednisolone alone without oral taper B. Oral prednisone 60 mg with two-week oral taper C. IV methylprednisolone for three days followed by oral prednisone taper D. Oral methylprednisolone (1 mg/kg per day) for three days then oral taper	A. 22% B. 32% C. 78% D. 92%

Question 9	Question 10
Which of the following are the characteristic demyelinating lesions on MRI for MS?	**Which of the following is the most likely prognosis for typical ON?**
A. Meningeal enhancement **B.** Suprasellar mass **C.** Ring-enhancing mass **D.** Multifocal periventricular white matter lesions	**A.** Full recovery in majority **B.** Partial recovery in majority **C.** Multiple recurrences without recovery **D.** Eventual no light perception vision

EXPLANATIONS

The solution to Question 1 is A.

Optic neuritis secondary to demyelinating disease typically presents with an acute to subacute (hours to days), unilateral vision loss and pain with eye movement. ON most commonly affects young Caucasian adults between 20 and 54 years old and is twice as prevalent in women as compared to men. Although ON is typically unilateral in the United States, bilateral ON can present more frequently in children and in non-North American/European patient populations (e.g., Asia, India, Africa).[1-7] In the Optic Neuritis Treatment Trial, the two most distinctive symptoms of ON in affected eyes were central vision loss (92.2%) and ocular or retro-orbital pain (92%), usually worsened by eye movement. The onset of eye pain commonly preceded or coincided with vision loss.[8] Although visual acuity varied greatly at presentation, the majority of patients recovered almost complete visual acuity and visual fields over a period of two months after presentation.[9,10] Although a unilateral ON typically presents with a detectable RAPD, an RAPD may not be present in a bilateral presentation due to the equal disruption in both afferent visual pathways. A detectable RAPD remained in one fourth of demyelinating ON patients up to two years later.[11]

The solution to Question 2 is B.

Two thirds of patients with typical Western demyelinating ON have retrobulbar optic neuritis with a normal-appearing optic nerve (Fig. 9.2). Only approximately one third of patients with acute ON have some degree of disc edema (papillitis) but when present the disc edema is typically mild. Other etiologies of optic neuropathy should be considered for atypical funduscopic findings (e.g., marked disc edema, peripapillary hemorrhages, or retinal exudates with a macular star figure) (Fig. 9.4). Optic neuropathies which could present as atypical demyelinating ON could include infectious (e.g., cat-scratch neuroretinitis), non-demyelinating inflammatory[12–14] (e.g., sarcoidosis), other autoimmune disorders (e.g., systemic lupus erythematosus), compressive lesions (e.g., meningioma), toxic (e.g., ethambutol), nutritional, ischemic (e.g., anterior ischemic optic neuropathy (AION)), and hereditary (e.g., Leber hereditary optic neuropathy

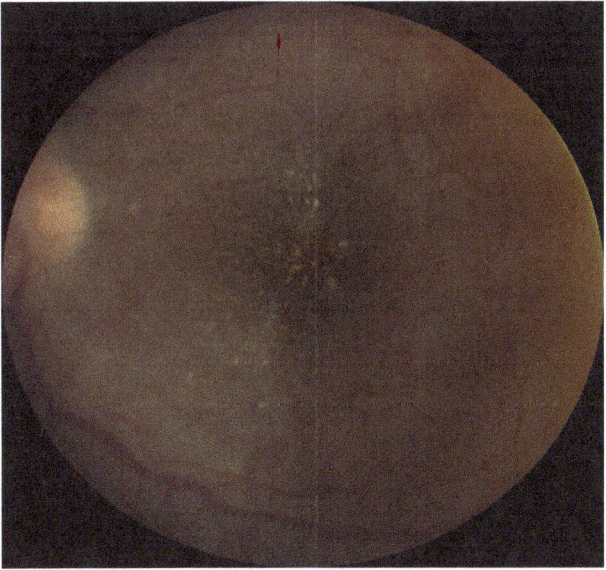

Fig. 9.4. Fundus photo showing atypical findings in ON, such as marked disc edema, peripapillary hemorrhages, retinal exudates, and a macular star figure. Other etiologies of optic neuropathy should be considered in these cases.

(LHON)).[15,16] Optic atrophy cannot be seen in the acute phase of ON but will develop over time (disc pallor), even after clinical recovery of each episode of ON.

The solution to Question 3 is B.

Assuming the presence of a bilateral optic neuropathy, the near reaction should be checked to detect any light-near dissociation (LND) OU.[17] Although efferent disease (e.g., Adie's tonic pupil) can produce LND, the loss of afferent signal in optic neuritis that is bilateral and symmetric can mask the presence of the RAPD and thus produce LND. Thus, the lack of a detectable RAPD does not exclude optic neuritis as the etiology for visual loss in bilateral cases. Formal visual field testing should also be performed to evaluate the severity and pattern of field loss because defects can vary from mild to severe, focal to diffuse, or involve only the central or peripheral field.

The solution to Question 4 is D.

ON visual field defects can be diffuse, nerve fiber bundle-related (altitudinal, arcuate), or involve the papillomacular bundle (cecocentral or central scotoma) (Fig. 9.5). Junctional visual field loss (junctional scotoma of Traquair) that is monocular and hemianopic is typically a compressive lesion and would be an atypical presentation for optic neuritis. A junctional scotoma (optic neuropathy in one eye and superotemporal field loss in the fellow eye), bitemporal hemianopsia, and homonymous hemianopsia involve the junction of the optic nerve and chiasm, the body of the chiasm, and the retrochiasmal pathway respectively and are not typical defects for ON. Regardless of the type of visual field defect in optic neuritis, most cases usually return to normal or near-normal visual function after recovery of acute ON.[17,18]

The solution to Question 5 is D.

MRI of the brain and orbits with gadolinium and fat saturation is the study of choice for the evaluation of an unexplained acute unilateral

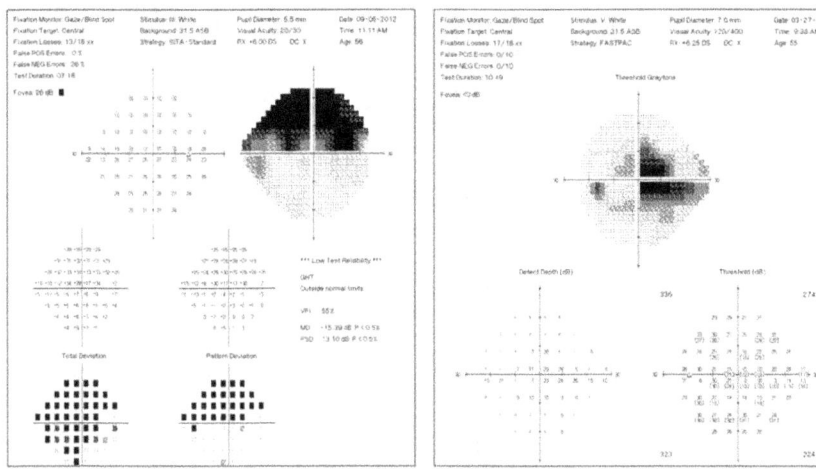

Fig. 9.5. Nerve fiber visual field defect seen in demyelinating ON. (a) Superior altitudinal VF defect, (b) cecocentral scotoma.

optic neuropathy in adults, including possible ON.[15,19] Non-enhanced (without gadolinium) MRI cannot judge lesion activity well, because demyelinating plaques in the acute phase are contrast enhancing. In addition, gadolinium is typically recommended because enhancement of the optic nerve is a distinctive and sensitive radiographic sign in the acute phase of ON and can involve the orbital or intracranial optic nerve. Optic nerve enhancement can be observed up to 8 to 12 weeks following acute demyelination and demyelinating white matter lesions are best seen on cranial MRI (especially T2 and FLAIR sequences) (Fig. 9.6). Thus, gadolinium-enhanced MRI can confirm the diagnosis of acute demyelinating ON and evaluate for additional demyelinating lesions. This information is an important prognostic indicator regarding the future risk of developing multiple sclerosis and is also used as baseline imaging to assess the patient's response to therapy.[20-24] Diffusion-weighted imaging (DWI) may be abnormal in demyelinating ON but is not specific or diagnostic and DWI is typically used for acute ischemic brain infarction. CT scan is not sensitive or specific for demyelinating white matter lesions when compared with MRI. CTA and magnetic

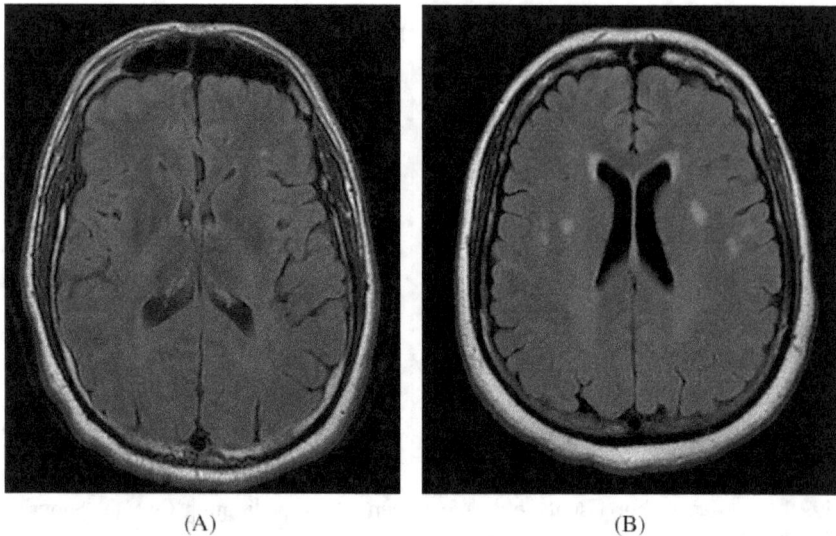

(A)   (B)

Fig. 9.6. Axial magnetic resonance imaging fluid-attenuated inversion recovery (FLAIR) sequence demonstrating periventricular white matter lesions typical of demyelination from multiple sclerosis. (A) Single white matter lesion. (B) Multiple white matter lesions.

resonance angiography (MRA) are angiographic studies used for evaluating vascular rather than demyelinating processes.

In atypical presentations of ON, other diagnoses must be excluded. Further workup is required to evaluate for MS mimics (e.g., sarcoidosis) or MS variants (e.g., neuromyelitis optica). In the ONTT the evaluation included laboratory testing (e.g., antinuclear antibody, syphilis serology, chest radiography) and a lumbar puncture. In typical cases these tests produced no new etiologies beyond demyelinating disease but testing may be warranted in atypical ON cases.

The solution to Question 6 is C.

Aquaporin-4-specific serum autoantibody has been recommended for recurrent or bilateral or non-recovering ON and in patients at risk for or suspected to have the variant of MS known as neuromyelitis optica, or Devic's disease,[25–27] who have had transverse myelitis.

Unilateral retrobulbar optic neuropathy in a young adult is a common presentation of typical idiopathic or demyelinating ON. The fundus finding of optic disc edema with a macular star figure is uncommon in demyelinating ON and is suggestive of infectious neuroretinitis (e.g., *Bartonella henselae*-related cat-scratch disease). We also consider NMO antibody in patients with long segments of enhancement of one or both optic nerves or chiasm on MRI especially when no classic demyelinating white matter lesions are seen.

The solution to Question 7 is C.

According to the Optic Neuritis Treatment Trial (a randomized, multicenter-controlled clinical trial), IV methylprednisolone followed by an oral taper is the preferred treatment for ON if faster visual recovery is desired. In the ONTT, patients were assigned to three groups: (1) oral prednisone (1 mg/kg of body weight per day) for 14 days; (2) IV methylprednisolone (1 g per day) for three days followed by oral prednisone (1 mg/kg/day) for 11 days; and (3) oral placebo for 14 days. The results showed that out of the three treatment arms, IV corticosteroids followed by an oral taper accelerated visual recovery, but did not improve the long-term visual outcome among treatment groups. Patients who were treated with oral corticosteroids alone had an increased rate of ON recurrence (30% recurrence rate at two years) when compared to placebo (16% recurrence rate) or IV methylprednisolone (13% recurrence rate). Although some practitioners use IV steroids alone this is not what was done in the ONTT and there might be some risk of deviating from the study protocol in the application of the results.[16,28]

The solution to Question 8 is C.

Due to the known association between ON and MS, the most important prognostic concern in patients with new-onset acute ON is the future risk of MS. The presence of characteristic demyelinating lesions on brain MRI is the strongest and most important predictor of developing MS. Over a 15-year observation period in the ONTT, patients presenting with an initial event of ON with a normal brain MRI had only a 25% risk of developing MS, compared to a 78% risk of developing MS if one or more lesions were present on brain MRI.[26,29–33]

The solution to Question 9 is D.

The characteristic demyelinating lesions observed on MRI are periventricular white matter plaques. The periventricular white matter is a favorite site for MS plaques. Periventricular plaques have an ovoid configuration, with the long axis oriented transversely. The ovoid lesions are termed Dawson's fingers for their finger-like appearance when observed on sagittal images involving the corpus callosum. Typical MS plaques have a homogeneous T2 MRI appearance with no cystic, hemorrhagic, or necrotic components (Fig. 9.6).

The solution to Question 10 is A.

Other prognostic concerns in patients with ON are visual recovery and the possibility of ON recurrence. Visual recovery is typically measured by visual acuity and/or visual field testing. Without treatment, the majority of patients improve after a few weeks. Visual improvement may continue over many months; 90% have 20/40 or better vision at one year.[8] Incomplete recovery is more often observed in patients with initially lower visual acuity, more severe visual field defects, or lesions of the optic nerve extending into the optic canal. However, in the ONTT, up to 64% of patients presenting with no light perception vision still recovered to a visual acuity of 20/40 or better.[10]

Recurrent ON is observed more frequently among individuals with a high risk for future MS development, or in MS variants such as neuromyelitis optica, or Devic's disease, especially in patients seropositive for the aquaporin-4-specific serum auto-antibody. African Americans have on average more severe visual loss at presentation (worse than 20/200),[26,29,31,34] with a worse prognosis for visual recovery as compared to Caucasian Americans.

SUMMARY

Optic neuritis secondary to demyelinating disease typically presents with an acute to subacute (hours to days), unilateral vision loss with pain that is worse upon eye movement. ON in the United States most commonly affects young Caucasian adults between 20 and 54 years old and is twice as prevalent in women as compared to men. Two thirds of patients with typical demyelinating ON have retrobulbar optic neuritis with a normal-appearing optic nerve. ON visual field defects can be diffuse, nerve fiber bundle-related (altitudinal, arcuate), or involve the papillomacular bundle (cecocentral or central scotoma) but are uncommonly monocular and hemianopic (junctional scotoma of Traquair). MRI of the brain and orbits with gadolinium and fat saturation is the study of choice for the evaluation of an unexplained acute optic neuropathy, including possible ON, but the main purpose of an MRI in ON is to evaluate for demyelinating disease and not to exclude alternative etiologies for the optic neuropathy. According to the ONTT, the best treatment for faster visual recovery is IV methylprednisolone for three days followed by oral prednisone for 11 days (14 days in total). The presence of characteristic demyelinating lesions on brain MRI is the strongest and most important predictor of developing MS. Over a 15-year observation period in the ONTT, patients presenting with an initial event of ON with a normal brain MRI had only a 25% risk of developing MS, compared to a 78% risk of developing MS if one or more lesions were present on brain MRI. Typical ON does not require additional laboratory testing or lumbar puncture for diagnosis but consideration for further evaluation should be made for atypical ON (including NMO).

REFERENCES

1. De la Cruz J, Kupersmith MJ. (2006) Clinical profile of simultaneous bilateral optic neuritis in adults. *Br J Ophthalmol* **90**:551–554.
2. Pokroy R, Modi G, Saffer D. (2001) Optic neuritis in an urban black African community. *Eye (Lond)* **15**:469–473.

3. Hwang JM, Lee YJ, Kim MK. (2002) Optic neuritis in Asian children. *J Pediatr Ophthalmol Strabismus* **39**:26–32.

4. Wang JC, Tow S, Aung T, *et al.* (2001) The presentation, aetiology, management and outcome of optic neuritis in an Asian population. *Clin Experiment Ophthalmol* **29**:312–315.

5. Lucchinetti CF, Kiers L, O'Duffy A, *et al.* (1997) Risk factors for developing multiple sclerosis after childhood optic neuritis. *Neurology* **49**:1413–1418.

6. Wilejto M, Shroff M, Buncic JR, *et al.* (2006) The clinical features, MRI findings, and outcome of optic neuritis in children. *Neurology* **67**:258–262.

7. Atkins EJ, Biousse V, Newman NJ. (2006) The natural history of optic neuritis. *Rev Neurol Dis* **3**:45–56.

8. The clinical profile of optic neuritis. Experience of the Optic Neuritis Treatment Trial. Optic Neuritis Study Group. (1991) *Arch Ophthalmol* **109**:1673–1678.

9. Celesia GG, Kaufman DI, Brigell M, *et al.* (1990) Optic neuritis: a prospective study. *Neurology* **40**:919–923.

10. Optic Neuritis Study Group. (1997) Visual function 5 years after optic neuritis: experience of the Optic Neuritis Treatment Trial. *Arch Ophthalmol* **115**:1545–1552.

11. Brusa A, Jones SJ, Plant GT. (2001) Long-term remyelination after optic neuritis: a 2-year visual evoked potential and psychophysical serial study. *Brain* **124**:468–479.

12. The clinical profile of optic neuritis. Experience of the Optic Neuritis Treatment Trial. Optic Neuritis Study Group. (1991) *Arch Ophthalmol* **109**:1673–1678.

13. Liu GT, Volpe NJ, Galetta S. eds. (2010) *Neuro-Ophthalmology: Diagnosis and Management*, 2nd ed. Elsevier, Philadelphia, PA.

14. Balcer LJ. (2006) Clinical practice. Optic neuritis. *N Engl J Med* **354**: 1273–1280.

15. Dooley MC, Foroozan R. (2010) Optic neuritis. *J Ophthalmic Vis Res* **5**: 182–187.

16. Pau D, Al Zubidi N, Yalamanchili S, *et al.* (2011) Optic neuritis. *Eye (Lond)* **25**:833–842.

17. Keltner JL, Johnson CA, Spurr JO, Beck RW. (1994) Visual field profile of optic neuritis. One-year follow-up in the Optic Neuritis Treatment Trial. *Arch Ophthalmol* **112**:946–953.

18. Beck RW, Gal RL, Bhatti MT, *et al.* (2004) Visual function more than 10 years after optic neuritis: experience of the optic neuritis treatment trial. *Am J Ophthalmol* **137**:77–83.

19. Optic Neuritis Study Group. (2008) Multiple sclerosis risk after optic neuritis: final optic neuritis treatment trial follow-up. *Arch Neurol* **65**:727–732.

20. Barker GJ. (2000) Technical issues for the study of the optic nerve with MRI. *J Neurol Sci* **172 Suppl 1**:S13–S16.

21. Jackson A, Sheppard S, Laitt RD, *et al.* (1998) Optic neuritis: MR imaging with combined fat- and water-suppression techniques. *Radiology* **206**:57–63.

22. Kupersmith MJ, Alban T, Zeiffer B, Lefton D. (2002) Contrast-enhanced MRI in acute optic neuritis: relationship to visual performance. *Brain* **125**:812–822.

23. Hickman SJ, Toosy AT, Miszkiel KA, *et al.* (2004) Visual recovery following acute optic neuritis—a clinical, electrophysiological and magnetic resonance imaging study. *J Neurol* **251**:996–1005.

24. He J, Grossman RI, Ge Y. (2001) Enhancing patterns in multiple sclerosis: evolution and persistence. *AJNR Am J Neuroradiol* **22**:664–669.

25. Pirko I, Blauwet LA, Blauwet LK, *et al.* (2004) The natural history of recurrent optic neuritis. *Arch Neurol* **61**:1401–1405.

26. Matiello M, Lennon VA, Jacob A, *et al.* (2008) NMO-IgG predicts the outcome of recurrent optic neuritis. *Neurology* **70**:2197–2200.

27. Petzold A, Pittock S, Lennon V, *et al.* (2010) Neuromyelitis optica-IgG (aquaporin-4) autoantibodies in immune mediated optic neuritis. *J Neurol Neurosurg Psychiatry* **81**:109–111.

28. Beck RW, Cleary PA, Anderson MM Jr, *et al.* (1992) A randomized, controlled trial of corticosteroids in the treatment of acute optic neuritis. The Optic Neuritis Study Group. *N Engl J Med* **326**:581–588.

29. Beck RW, Trobe JD, Moke PS, *et al.* (2003) High- and low-risk profiles for the development of multiple sclerosis within 10 years after optic neuritis: experience of the optic neuritis treatment trial. *Arch Ophthalmol* **121**:944–949.

30. Nilsson P, Larsson EM, Maly-Sundgren P, *et al.* (2005) Predicting the outcome of optic neuritis: evaluation of risk factors after 30 years of follow-up. *J Neurol* **252**:396–402.

31. Banwell B, Tenembaum S, Lennon VA, *et al.* (2008) Neuromyelitis optica-IgG in childhood inflammatory demyelinating CNS disorders. *Neurology* **70**:344–352.

32. The 5-year risk of MS after optic neuritis. Experience of the optic neuritis treatment trial. Optic Neuritis Study Group. (1997) *Neurology* **49**:1404–1413.

33. Optic Neuritis Study Group. (2008) Multiple sclerosis risk after optic neuritis: final optic neuritis treatment trial follow-up. *Arch Neurol* **65**:727–732.

34. Phillips PH, Newman NJ, Lynn MJ. (1998) Optic neuritis in African Americans. *Arch Neurol* **55**:186–192.

10

Third Nerve Palsy

Arielle Spitze MD, Rabeea Khan MD, Nagham Al-Zubidi MD, Sushma Yalamanchili MD, and Andrew G. Lee MD

CASE

A 79-year-old Caucasian man presented with a four-day history of left retrobulbar pain and a left-sided headache which he described as 10/10 in severity and throbbing in quality. One day later, he developed diplopia and left upper lid ptosis. His past medical history was significant for stage III colorectal adenocarcinoma, for which he had a colorectal resection and received chemotherapy and radiation therapy. He had prior coronary artery disease treated with coronary artery bypass. His medications included aspirin, clopidogrel, metoprolol, ramipril, niacin, and donepezil. He smoked cigarettes in the distant past but denied any alcohol or illicit drug use. There was no temporal artery tenderness or nodularity. Best-corrected visual acuity was 20/25+1 in the right eye (OD) and 20/30−1 in the left eye (OS). Extraocular motility was full OD, but revealed a 25-prism-diopter left exotropia (XT) in primary gaze with −4 limitation of adduction, −3 underaction of supraduction and infraduction, but full abduction OS (see Fig. 10.1). There was intorsion in downgaze suggesting an intact fourth nerve. There was no trigeminal or facial nerve dysfunction. Confrontation visual field testing was full in both eyes (OU). Automated Humphrey visual fields (24-2) showed non-specific scatter OD and left superior lid artifact from the left ptosis. There was no variability or fatigue, Cogan's lid twitch sign, or enhancement of ptosis. Pupils were both reactive and measured 3 mm in the dark and 1 mm in the light OU with no relative afferent pupillary defect

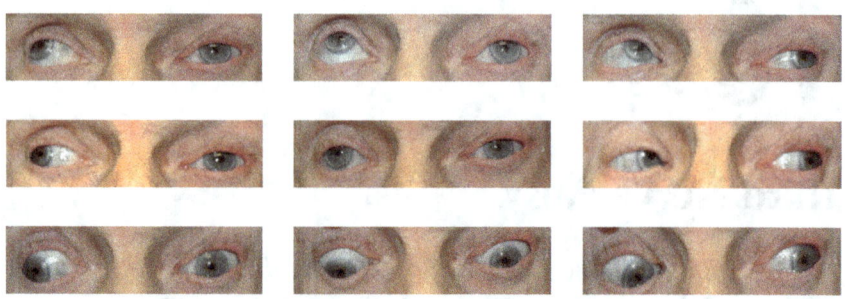

Fig. 10.1. Montage of extraocular motility in the nine gaze positions in a patient with pupil-sparing left cranial nerve III palsy. Please note that although the patient was not able to open his left upper lid, it was being held open by an assistant for these photographs.

(RAPD) or anisocoria. Slit lamp exam was significant for corneal arcus OU, and 2+ nuclear sclerotic cataracts OU consistent with 20/30 vision OU. Fundus examination was within normal limits OU. There was no optic disc edema or optic atrophy OU.

Cranial computed tomography (CT) and CT angiography (CTA) were both negative and no aneurysm was seen. Erythrocyte sedimentation rate (ESR) was 55 mm/hr and C-reactive protein (CRP) was 2.3 mg/L. The patient was then started on 1 g of IV methylprednisolone for possible giant cell arteritis; however, temporal artery biopsy was negative for gaint cell arteritis. Magnetic resonance imaging (MRI) of the brain and orbits and MR angiography (MRA) of the brain and neck showed subtle enhancement of the left anterior clinoid and cavernous sinus (Fig. 10.2). Positron emission tomography (PET) showed presumed metastatic lesions to the thoracic and lumbar spine which were biopsied and positive for metastatic colon adenocarcinoma. The patient returned to oncology for systemic chemotherapy.

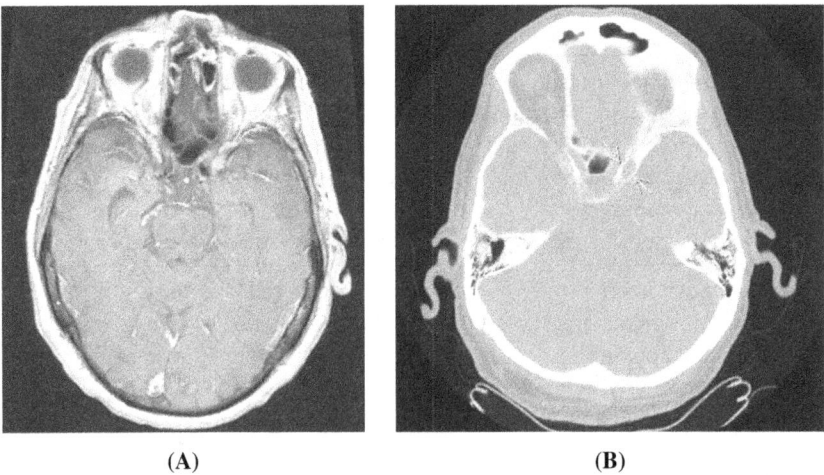

(A)   (B)

Fig. 10.2. MRI of the brain and orbits (A) which demonstrated subtle enhancement of the left anterior clinoid and cavernous sinus and CT (B) demonstrating a lytic appearance of the left anterior clinoid lesion.

Question 1	Question 2
Which of the following is the most likely cause of an acute, neurologically isolated, pupil-sparing, complete third nerve palsy in a 75 year-old diabetic man?	Which of the following is the most likely pupillary finding in an acute, isolated, complete third nerve palsy due to an aneurysm?
A. Ischemia B. Neoplasm C. Myasthenia gravis D. Aneurysm	A. Ipsilateral pupillary miosis B. Relative afferent pupillary defect C. Light-near dissociation D. Ipsilateral mydriasis

Question 3	Question 4
In a 30-year-old patient with an acute third nerve palsy, the fundus findings shown in Fig 10.3 would most likely suggest which of the following diagnoses?	In a 47-year-old previously healthy and immunocompetent patient who presents with an acute third nerve palsy, hypotension, lethargy, fever, and sudden vision loss, which of the following is the most likely diagnosis?
A. Giant cell arteritis **B.** Increased intracranial pressure **C.** Pituitary apoplexy **D.** Unruptured posterior communicating artery aneurysm	**A.** Giant cell arteritis **B.** Ophthalmoplegic migraine **C.** Orbital apex Mucor **D.** Pituitary apoplexy
Question 5	**Question 6**
A 70-year-old man presents with scalp tenderness, jaw claudication, and a pupil-sparing left third nerve palsy. Which of the following is the most appropriate initial step?	An aneurysm of which of the following arteries is most likely to produce an acute, pupil-involved third nerve palsy?
A. Temporal artery biopsy **B.** Stat ESR and CRP **C.** CTA of the head **D.** MRI of the head	**A.** Anterior communicating artery **B.** Posterior inferior cerebellar artery **C.** Posterior communicating artery **D.** Posterior cerebral artery
Question 7	**Question 8**
A lesion at which of the following locations is most likely to produce a nuclear third nerve palsy?	Which of the following would be the required initial imaging study for a neurologically isolated, painless, acute, pupil-sparing, unilateral third cranial nerve palsy in a hypertensive and diabetic patient?
A. Medulla **B.** Pons **C.** Midbrain **D.** Thalamus	**A.** CT of the head **B.** MRI of the orbit followed by cerebral angiography **C.** MRI of the head without contrast **D.** No imaging necessary if improving

Question 9	Question 10
Which of the following is the most beneficial initial treatment for a presumed ischemic, acute, isolated cranial nerve III palsy present for one week?	**Which of the following is the most likely outcome from an isolated, presumed vasculopathic cranial nerve III palsy?**
A. Patching of the affected eye **B.** Injection of botulinum toxin **C.** Lateral rectus recession **D.** Superior oblique tendon transposition	**A.** Continued worsening requiring strabismus surgery **B.** Spontaneous recovery after six to eight weeks **C.** Aberrant regeneration of lid, motility, or pupil **D.** Painful torticollis from chronic head tilt

EXPLANATIONS

The solution to Question 1 is A.

Third nerve palsies represent up to 30% of all cranial nerve palsies in adults[1] and microvascular ischemia is the underlying etiology in 17–35% of retrospective pooled series.[1] Although ischemia is the most common etiology, compressive lesions (e.g., aneurysm and neoplasm) are responsible for up to 19% of cases of third nerve palsy. The most common location of an aneurysm producing a third nerve palsy is the posterior communicating artery–internal carotid artery junction (34–61% of cases), but basilar tip aneurysms and intracavernous internal carotid artery aneurysms can also produce a unilateral or bilateral third nerve palsy. Thus, the common initial imaging study for patients suspected of harboring an aneurysm is a cranial CT (noncontrast) for subarachnoid hemorrhage, especially in the emergency room setting or in patients with severe pain (e.g., "worst headache of my life"). The CT can then be followed with a contrast CT/cranial angiography (CTA) for aneurysm (cranial CT/CTA). Unfortunately, cranial CT/CTA is not sufficient for excluding non-aneurysmal causes of third nerve palsy and a cranial/orbital MRI and MRA with and without contrast might still be necessary in an unexplained third nerve palsy. Although meningiomas and other benign cavernous sinus lesions can produce a third nerve palsy, metastatic neoplasm should be suspected in patients with acute presentations or in known cancer patients (as in this case). Myasthenia gravis should also be considered in any painless, pupil-sparing ophthalmoplegia including what might appear to be a typical third nerve palsy. Pituitary adenomas with cavernous extension (e.g., pituitary apoplexy) and other less common neoplastic etiologies (e.g., third nerve schwannoma, intracavernous hemangioma/ hemangiopericytoma) or vascular lesions (e.g., intracavernous aneurysm, carotid-cavernous fistula) may also produce a third nerve palsy. Giant cell arteritis should also be considered in the differential diagnosis of any new diplopia in elderly patients, especially those with headache, jaw pain, or visual loss. Trauma is an uncommon but typically obvious cause of a third nerve palsy and in pooled retrospective series comprises less than 1% of cases.[1]

In this patient, the cavernous sinus mass in the setting of known stage III adenocarcinoma of the colon triggered a metastatic evaluation with PET scan for an alternative source to biopsy, which ultimately led to confirmation of metastatic disease.

The solution to Question 2 is D.

The third cranial nerve carries the parasympathetic fibers to the iris sphincter of the pupil from the Edinger–Westphal nucleus in the dorsal midbrain and also the somatic ocular motor fibers that innervate the inferior oblique, medial rectus, superior rectus, inferior rectus, and levator palpebrae superioris muscles.[1] A complete loss of third nerve function results in unopposed action of the lateral rectus muscle (innervated by the sixth cranial nerve) and the superior oblique muscle (innervated by the fourth cranial nerve). This results in the classic presentation in a third nerve palsy of an eye that is "down and out" (i.e., in the abducted and depressed position.[1] Additionally, partial or complete ptosis results from lack of levator palpebrae superioris function, and a poorly reactive or non-reactive pupil with anisocoria results from loss of parasympathetic iris sphincter innervation. This produces an anisocoria that is greater in the light. The lid, pupil, or muscle function might be variably involved or spared in partial third nerve palsies. In contrast, miosis, ptosis, anisocoria greater in the dark (from poor pupillary dilation with dilation lag), and anhidrosis are seen in Horner syndrome, which results from interruption of the ocular sympathetic outflow tract. Horner syndrome produces only a mild ptosis (from involvement of the sympathetically innervated Müller muscle); therefore, a complete or nearly complete ptosis with aniso-coria greater in the light should suggest concomitant third nerve palsy with Horner syndrome (e.g., cavernous sinus localization). In addition, in the chronic phase of a compressive or traumatic third nerve palsy, the pupil may become miotic over time due to aberrant regeneration. In the acute setting, however, the pupil in a typical pupil-involved third nerve palsy is dilated and poorly reactive rather than miotic. A RAPD is seen when there is damage to the afferent input from the retina/optic nerve to the pretectal midbrain and third nerve nucleus. A RAPD would not be seen in an efferent problem alone such as third nerve palsy, but might rarely occur without visual loss from dorsal midbrain involvement of the pretectal interneuron (i.e., a tectal RAPD). Acute visual loss with a RAPD suggests an ipsilateral concomitant optic neuropathy and in the setting of a third nerve palsy is suggestive of ipsilateral orbital apex involvement or less likely multiple (e.g., metastatic) lesions or a systemic (e.g., giant cell arteritis) process.

The solution to Question 3 is B.

In a patient with an acute third nerve palsy and associated bilateral papilledema (see Fig. 10.3), a lesion producing increased intracranial pressure should be suspected. The third nerve may be involved in uncal herniation from an expanding mass lesion in which the uncus, located in the medial portion of the temporal lobe, herniates through the foramen magnum, directly compressing the third cranial nerve at the tentorium and causing a third nerve palsy. The dilated and poorly

Right eye   Left eye

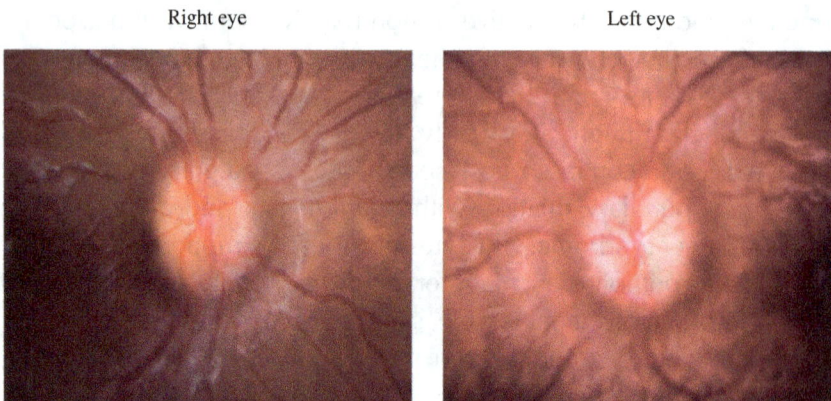

Fig. 10.3. Photos of bilateral disc edema in a patient with increased intracranial pressure, or papilledema.

reactive pupil associated with uncal herniation is sometimes known as a Hutchinson pupil[1] and is a false localizing sign. Lesions producing uncal herniation may result in obstruction of cerebrospinal fluid outflow, causing elevated intracranial pressure which can manifest as papilledema. A ruptured posterior communicating artery aneurysm could also cause increased intracranial pressure from hemorrhage and secondary papilledema, but imaging would differentiate this etiology. An unruptured aneurysm might produce a painful, pupil-involved third nerve palsy but would not be expected to produce papilledema. Although pituitary apoplexy can produce unilateral (i.e., optic neuropathy) or bilateral (e.g., bitemporal hemianopsia) visual loss in addition to a third nerve palsy (due to cavernous sinus extension), papilledema would not be expected in pituitary apoplexy. Although papilledema is a distinctive sign of pseudotumor cerebri, unlike a non-localizing sixth nerve palsy, a third nerve palsy is not a common finding in idiopathic intracranial hypertension. Further imaging and testing in this circumstance is warranted (e.g., contrast cranial MRI/magnetic resonance venography and lumbar puncture).

The solution to Question 4 is D.

Pituitary apoplexy results from acute hemorrhage or necrosis occurring within a pre-existing pituitary adenoma, which causes rapid enlargement of the pituitary gland and compression of the surrounding structures. The most common structures involved in apoplexy are the cavernous sinus (which may result in an acute third nerve palsy) and the optic nerves or chiasm, resulting in loss of vision unilaterally or bilaterally (junctional visual field loss or bitemporal hemianopsia). Cardiovascular instability, lethargy, and fever can result from the lack of adrenocorticotropic hormone release from the non-functioning pituitary gland (i.e., Addisonian crisis) and can be life-threatening.[1] Although giant cell arteritis (GCA) can present with sudden vision loss, lethargy, and fever, hypotension is not a typical feature and GCA is a disease of elderly (> 50 years old) patients. Third nerve palsies associated with GCA are rare but have been reported and therefore GCA remains in the differential diagnosis of diplopia in the elderly. Older patients should be specifically questioned about typical symptoms of GCA and if indicated, laboratory (e.g., ESR and CRP) and other procedures (i.e., temporal artery biopsy) might be necessary.[1] An ophthalmoplegic migraine is characterized by recurrent bouts of a third cranial nerve (or rarely other ocular motor cranial nerve) palsy in the setting of a younger patient with migraine.[2] Ophthalmoplegic migraines are a diagnosis of exclusion and typically cranial contrast MRI with MRA as well as other testing (laboratory, lumbar puncture) are necessary to exclude other etiologies. Orbital apex fungal disease would be in the differential diagnosis of ipsilateral visual loss (due to concomitant optic neuropathy), proptosis, and a third nerve palsy (or any degree of ophthalmoplegia), but mucormycosis is typically a disease of immunosuppressed individuals, particularly diabetic patients in diabetic ketoacidosis. Although optic disc edema can occur ipsilaterally, bilateral optic disc edema would be atypical for "mucormycosis". CT scan of the orbit/sinuses and head should differentiate sinus-based fungal disease with extension to the orbital apex from pituitary apoplexy with cavernous sinus extension.

The solution to Question 5 is B.

Although GCA typically presents with unilateral or bilateral visual loss (often with pallid optic disc edema), it can also produce diplopia in elderly patients. The serum erythrocyte sedimentation rate and C-reactive protein are acute biomarkers of systemic inflammation that are typically elevated in GCA and we order them stat for our emergent patients with GCA.[4] Empiric high-dose oral or intravenous corticosteroids should be initiated once the diagnosis of GCA is considered, although a temporal artery biopsy is often need for diagnostic confirmation.[4] The serum CRP in combination with ESR has greater sensitivity for GCA than the ESR or CRP alone and we recommend that the combination of the two acute-phase reactants be performed in suspected GCA.[4] However, the temporal artery biopsy still remains the gold standard for the definitive diagnosis of GCA.

The solution to Question 6 is C.

The most common aneurysm causing an acute, unilateral third nerve palsy is an aneurysm of the posterior communicating artery (PCommA) and internal carotid artery junction. The anatomic course of the third nerve originates from the third nerve nucleus and fasicle located in the midbrain. The nerve exits ventrally, travels anteriorly to the cavernous sinus, and closely parallels the PCommA in the subarachnoid space.[1] The pupillary fibers are located within the most superficial layers of the subarachnoid portion of the third cranial nerve. Thus, ipsilateral compression by a PCommA aneurysm typically causes pupillary involvement. In contrast, diabetic (and other small vessel ischemic etiologic) third nerve palsies often spare the pupil, as ischemia involves the deeper penetrating vasa nervorum vessels and spares the superficial pupillary fibers. Some diabetic ischemic third nerve palsies however do involve the pupil (albeit with mild < 1 mm of anisocoria). Occasionally, aneurysms of the basilar tip or anterior choroidal artery may cause third nerve palsies, but an aneurysm of the PCommA is the most common cause of an aneurysmal third nerve palsy.[1] Aneurysms of the posterior inferior cerebellar (PICA) and posterior cerebral arteries (PCA) are not typically associated with a third nerve palsy. A PICA infarct can produce a Wallenberg syndrome which can manifest as a Horner syndrome or torsional nystagmus. A PCA infarct can produce a contralateral homonymous hemianopsia.

Although the "rule of the pupil" states that a pupil-involving third nerve palsy is a PCommA aneurysm until proven otherwise, the absence of pupil involvement does not rule out a PCommA aneurysm; up to 33% of all PCommA aneurysms do not have pupillary involvement on presentation.[1] In some cases, the pupil is not involved because of partial involvement of the third cranial nerve (e.g., partial palsy or superior division only) and thus the "rule of the pupil" should not be extrapolated to clinically define "pupil-sparing" in partial third nerve palsies. Conversely, diabetic ischemic third nerve palsy typically presents as an isolated, pupil-sparing (i.e., pupil function completely normal) but otherwise complete third nerve palsy, albeit some diabetic palsies can have minimal (< 1 mm) anisocoria.

The solution to Question 7 is C.

All of the ocular motor cranial nerves (III, IV, VI) originate in the brainstem.[5] The dorsal midbrain contains the nuclei and fascicles for cranial nerves III (at the level of the superior colliculus) and IV (at the level of the inferior colliculus).[5] The dorsal pons contains the nuclei for cranial nerve VI.[5] The medulla contains the lower cranial nerves, including IX, X, XI, and XII, but not the ocular motor cranial nerves.[5] The thalamus and thalamo-mesencephalic junction have connections to the brainstem, controlling supranuclear gaze, but do not contain the ocular motor nuclei or their fascicles or nerves.

The solution to Question 8 is D.

Although this is somewhat controversial, a complete, isolated, acute, painless third nerve palsy in a vasculopathic patient without pupillary involvement could be observed for improvement, as microvascular ischemia is the most likely culprit.[6] Other authors, however, believe that the clinical features of third nerve palsy are not sufficient to differentiate an aneurysm and that all patients regardless of pupil involvement or sparing should undergo a CTA as an initial study. In contrast, for a third nerve palsy with a "blown" (dilated) pupil, the pre-test likelihood for aneurysm is high and thus a CT/CTA would be recommended followed by a contrast MRI/MRA to rule out non-aneurysmal causes of third nerve palsy. Although CTA is believed to be superior to MRA at most centers, variability in technique, availability of neuroradiologic interpretation, and sometimes the intrinsic imaging characteristics of the aneurysm itself (e.g., thrombosis, partial flow) might make one technique better than the other in any one individual patient. Specific, customized, individualized discussion and review of the neuroimaging studies with the neuroradiologist is recommended.[6] Even though both MRA and CTA have a sensitivity of close to 98% for the detection of an aneurysm producing a third nerve palsy, structural MRI with contrast can better detect non-aneurysmal causes of third nerve palsy (e.g., tumor, meningeal disease).[6] Catheter contrast angiography (CA) should be considered even if the MRI/CT and MRA/CTA combination is negative for aneurysm if there is sufficiently high pretest (e.g., painful, pupil-involved third nerve palsy) or post-test (CTA/MRA) likelihood of aneurysm (e.g., CTA or MRA had artifact obscuring a complete three-dimensional rotational view of the PCommA).[6] Both combinationns of a complete third nerve palsy with partial pupillary involvement and partial third nerve palsy without pupillary involvement typically require some type of imaging study (e.g., CT/CTA then MRI /MRA).[6] However, CA may not be necessary in such cases if the index of suspicion is not as high for aneurysm after adequate non-catheter cranial and cerebrovascular imaging. CT or MRI of the orbits alone would not be the imaging study of choice for a third nerve palsy because the course of the third nerve has both intracranial and intraorbital components. MRI without contrast is not recommended because enhancing lesions of the third cranial nerve will be missed without gadolinium contrast. Some patients, however, have contraindications (e.g., renal failure, allergy) that might preclude contrast administration. MRA (as opposed to contrast CTA) can be performed with or without contrast and a non-contrast MRA might be a reasonable alternative in selected cases with contrast contraindications. Although we believe that initial observation without neuroimaging is a reasonable practice option for an acute, isolated, painless, pupil-sparing third nerve palsy in a vasculo-pathic patient, the development of pain, progression, lack of improvement, aberrant regeneration, or any new neurologic signs or symptoms during the observation period (i.e., first few weeks) should prompt consideration for neuroimaging. On the other hand, MRI/MRA with and without contrast of the head is safe and would not be unreasonable even in cases of acute, isolated, painless, pupil-sparing, and presumed vasculopathic third nerve palsy because some of these patients are harboring an underlying etiology. However, the decision to image in this setting remains controversial because most cases that have a lesion as the underlying etiology would eventually come to neuroimaging because of lack of spontaneous improvement.

The solution to Question 9 is A.

Patching of the affected eye and the use of temporary Fresnel prisms are first-line treatments for an acute cranial nerve three palsy, as they are both non-invasive and reversible. Use of grind-in prism is gener-ally not recommended in the acute phase because patients may continue to worsen or improve and the amount of prism might need to be changed. Surgical treatment should be considered only after the diagnostic evaluation is completed. If the deviation fails to improve, fails conservative or prismatic therapy, and the orthoptic measurements have remained stable for at least several months, then strabismus surgery could be considered.[1] Surgical correction of third nerve palsy-related ptosis and strabismus is notoriously difficult. The precise surgical procedures selected of course depend on the exact pattern of strabismus. Commonly employed procedures to alleviate symptomatic diplopia including transposition of the superior oblique tendon, medial rectus resection, and lateral rectus recession.[7] The efficacy of botulinum toxin injection in the treatment of an acute third nerve palsy is controversial, but has been shown to allow medial rectus recovery by relaxing the lateral rectus muscle.[8,9] Botulinum toxin can also be effective in temporarily treating symptomatic diplopia if the patient is not ready to proceed with more permanent surgical procedures.

The solution to Question 10 is B.

Almost half of all idiopathic third cranial nerve palsies resolve partially or completely[1] and a presumed vasculopathic cranial nerve three palsy has an even higher rate of spontaneous resolution, with up to 80% resolving in three months.[10] As a result, in contrast to longstanding deviations that might produce an anomalous head or face position, ischemic third nerve palsy typically would not result in painful torticollis. Multiple simultaneous or rapidly sequential cranial neuropathies are atypical and should prompt further evaluation for additional diagnoses including neuroimaging (i.e., a diabetic patient is allowed only one ocular motor cranial neuropathy at a time). Aberrant regeneration is essentially never seen after ischemic third nerve palsy and thus if aberrant regeneration is present, this should prompt neuroimaging, including evaluation for neoplasm (especially cavernous sinus) or aneurysm.[1]

SUMMARY

An acute, unilateral, painless, pupil-sparing third nerve palsy is most often caused by microvascular ischemia in adults. Some cases, however, (especially pupil-involving third nerve palsies) are produced by aneurysms (most commonly of the PCommA), inflammation, infection, or neoplasms; thus, consideration for neuroimaging should be made in every patient (e.g., CT/CTA and MRI/MRA). A complete pupil-involving third nerve palsy includes complete ptosis, an eye that is "down and out" (i.e., ipsilateral exotropia and hypotropia), and a poorly or non-reactive pupil with anisocoria greater in the light. Third nerve palsies, however, do not have to be complete (i.e., partial third nerve palsy) and do not have to involve the pupil (i.e., pupil-sparing third nerve palsy). An acute third nerve palsy with a "blown" (dilated) pupil in the intensive care unit setting, especially in patients with increased intracranial pressure, is an ominous sign of acute neurologic decompensation and typically requires an emergent cranial CT scan. Acute, painful third nerve palsy due to pituitary apoplexy is an emergency that may or may not be associated with concomitant compression of the optic chiasm, and systemic symptoms and signs including cardiovascular instability, lethargy, or fever. GCA rarely causes a third nerve palsy but should be considered in elderly patients who present with diplopia with or without visual loss, headache, jaw claudication, or other symptoms of GCA. In any third nerve palsy, but particularly in pupil-involving cases, an aneurysm of the PCommA should be considered to be the underlying etiology until proven otherwise (the "rule of the pupil"). The lack of pupillary involvement in a partial third nerve palsy, however, does not obviate the need to rule out a PCommA aneurysm, as up to 33% of all PCommA aneurysms do not have pupillary involvement on presentation. Typically, the best initial imaging studies are cranial CT/contrast CTA but MRI/MRA with and without contrast might still be necessary to exclude other non-aneurysmal causes of third nerve palsy. Myasthenia gravis should also be considered in any painless, pupil-sparing ophthal-moplegia, including what appears to be a typical third nerve palsy. Although this is controversial, an acute, complete, isolated third nerve palsy without pupillary involvement in a vasculopathic patient can be observed for spontaneous improvement, but lack of improvement, progression, or development of aberrant regeneration should prompt neuroimaging. Patching and/or temporary Fresnel prisms are common first-line treatments for stable cranial nerve III palsies but strabismus and/or ptosis surgery may be necessary for chronic and stable cases.

REFERENCES

1. Rucker JC. (2012) Diplopia, third nerve palsies, and sixth nerve palsies. In: Roos KL (ed), *Emergency Neurology*. Springer, New York, NY, pp. 113–132.
2. Margari L, Legrottaglie AR, Craig F, *et al.* (2012) Ophthalmoplegic migraine: migraine or oculomotor neuropathy? *Cephalgia* **32**:1208–1215.
3. Pugh MB, ed. (2006) *Stedman's Medical Dictionary*, 28th ed. Lippincott Williams & Wilkins, Baltimore, MD.
4. Kermani TA, Schmidt J, Crowson CS, *et al.* (2012) Utility of erythrocyte sedimentation rate and C-reactive protein for the diagnosis of giant cell arteritis. *Semin Arthritis Rheum* **41**:866–871.
5. Hendelman W. (2006) *Atlas of Functional Neuroanatomy*. CRC Press, Boca Raton, FL.
6. Lee AG, Johnson MC, Policeni BA, Smoker WR. (2009) Imaging for neuro-ophthalmic and orbital disease — a review. *Clin Experiment Ophthalmol* **37**:30–53.
7. Yonghong J, Kanxing Z, Wei L, *et al.* (2008) Surgical management of large-angle incomitant strabismus in patients with oculomotor nerve palsy. *JAAPOS* **12**:49–53.
8. Metz HS, Mazow M. (1988) Botulinum toxin treatment of acute sixth and third nerve palsy. *Graefes Arch Clin Exp Ophthalmol* **226**:141–144.
9. Rowe FJ, Noonan CP. (2012) Botulinum toxin for the treatment of strabismus. *Cochrane Database Syst Rev* **2**:CD006499.
10. Akagi T, Miyamoto K, Kashii S, Yoshimura N. (2008) Cause and prognosis of neurologically isolated third, fourth, or sixth cranial nerve dysfunction in cases of oculomotor palsy. *Jpn J Ophthalmol* **52**:32–35.

11

Fourth Nerve Palsy

*Arielle Spitze MD, Jason Zhang BA, Nagham Al-Zubidi MD,
Sushma Yalamanchili MD, and Andrew G. Lee MD*

CASE

A 69-year-old Caucasian male presented to the emergency room with acute-onset severe frontal headache, nausea, and acute, binocular diplopia. Past medical history was significant for hypertension, type II diabetes, hyperlipidemia, and an ischemic stroke 10 years prior. The initial blood pressure measured 199/97 mmHg. Computed tomography (CT) of the head without contrast (performed first) and with contrast showed no acute intracranial abnormalities. A subsequent cranial magnetic resonance imaging (MRI) scan with and without contrast was unremarkable except for age-related small vessel ischemic changes. The patient denied any symptoms of giant cell arteritis (e.g., scalp tenderness, temporal nodularity, or jaw claudication), history of eye trauma, strabismus surgery, or lazy eye. Laboratory studies including erythrocyte sedimentation rate (ESR), C-reactive protein (CRP), hemoglobin/hematocrit, thyroid-stimulating hormone (TSH), free T3, and free T4 were all within normal limits. Serum glucose was elevated at 154 mg/dL and hemoglobin A1c was elevated at 8.83%. Serum cholesterol and triglycerides were elevated at 194 mg/dL and 179 mg/dL, respectively. The remainder of the medical history was negative. The patient remained in the emergency room until his blood pressure was stabilized. Upon discharge, he was referred to the outpatient neuro-ophthalmology service for evaluation.

On neuro-ophthalmologic examination, the patient's best-corrected visual acuity was 20/25 in the right eye (OD) and 20/30 in the left eye (OS). Pupils were 4 mm in the dark and 3 mm in the light with no relative afferent pupillary defect (RAPD). External examination showed a subtle left head tilt of 5 degrees. There was no scalp tenderness or temporal artery nodularity. Motility examination revealed a 10-prism-diopter (PD) right hypertropia (RHT) in primary gaze, a 5 PD RHT in right gaze, a 14 PD RHT in left gaze, a 4 PD RHT in upgaze, and an 8 PD RHT with 3 PD esotropia (ET) in downgaze (see Fig. 11.1). On right head tilt there was a 12 PD RHT while on left head tilt an 8 PD RHT was observed. Double Maddox rod testing showed 5 degrees of excyclotorsion OD. Intraocular pressure measurements, slit lamp biomicroscopy, visual field testing, and ophthalmoscopic examinations were all normal in both eyes (OU). The patient was instructed to wear a patch on his right eye for symptomatic relief and to follow up with his primary care physician for management of his hypertension, hyperlipidemia, and diabetes. He returned six weeks later and had complete resolution of his diplopia at that time.

	4^ΔRHT	
5^ΔRHT	10^ΔRHT	14^ΔRHT
	8^ΔRHT, 3^ΔET	

Right Head Tilt: 12^ΔRHT
Left Head Tilt: 8^ΔRHT

Fig. 11.1. Gaze examination of the right eye indicated a 10-prism-diopter right hypertropia in primary gaze that worsened in left gaze and right head tilt, consistent with a right fourth nerve palsy. Because the superior oblique has an abducting function in downgaze, an esotropia will often be more likely to manifest in that position, as demonstrated in the measurements.

Question 1	Question 2
Which of the following arteries is most likely to harbor an aneurysm producing an isolated fourth nerve palsy?	Which of the following findings is most likely to be present in a right fourth nerve palsy?
A. Anterior communicating artery B. Posterior communicating artery C. Superior cerebellar artery D. Vertebral artery	A. Right head tilt B. Right hypotropia C. Right hypoglobus D. Right excyclotorsion
Question 3	Question 4
Which of the following tests is the most useful in detecting ocular cyclotorsion?	Which of the following findings is most characteristic of a bilateral fourth nerve palsy?
A. Hirschberg test B. Cover-uncover test C. Dilated funduscopic examination D. Single Maddox rod test	A. Large vertical deviation in primary gaze B. Right hypertropia in right gaze and left hypertropia in left gaze C. V-pattern exotropia in downgaze D. More than 10 degrees of excyclotorsion
Question 5	Question 6
Which of the following ocular deviations is most consistent with a positive three-step Bielschowsky test for a right fourth nerve palsy?	In an adult patient presenting with a neurologically isolated, acute, unilateral fourth nerve palsy, which of the following is the most common etiology?
A. Right hypertropia worse on right head tilt B. Right hypertropia worse on left head tilt C. Right hypotropia worse on left head tilt D. Right hypotropia worse on right head tilt	A. Myasthenia gravis B. Midbrain infarction C. Head trauma D. Systemic vasculitis

Question 7	Question 8
An adult patient with a fourth nerve palsy complains of chronic neck pain and brings childhood photographs showing a longstanding right head tilt. Which of the following best describes the etiology of her cranial nerve deficit?	A patient with an isolated presumed vasculopathic right fourth nerve palsy returns three months later with an increased right hypertropia in all positions of gaze. What is the best next step in management?
A. Intracranial hypertension B. Congenital, decompensated C. Neoplastic midbrain lesion D. Post-infectious	A. Start a regimen of empiric low-dose PO corticosteroids B. B-scan ultrasonography of the right eye C. MRI of the brain and orbits with and without contrast with fat suppression D. Refer the patient to a strabismus surgeon

EXPLANATIONS

The solution to Question 1 is C.

The fourth cranial nerve (trochlear nerve) nucleus lies caudal to the oculomotor nucleus and dorsal to the medial longitudinal fasciculus within the midbrain.[1,2] The fourth nerve first travels inferiorly and then posteriorly around the cerebral aqueduct, decussating at the anterior medullary velum before emerging just below the inferior colliculi.[3] Within the subarachnoid space, it then passes between the posterior cerebral artery and the superior cerebellar artery, where it is most vulnerable to possible aneurysmal compression (answer choice C), although this is an unusual cause of fourth nerve palsy. The fourth nerve then continues along the undersurface of the tentorial edge of the tentorium cerebelli before piercing the dura and entering the lateral wall of the cavernous sinus. The nerve then enters the orbit through the superior orbital fissure to innervate the superior oblique muscle. Aneurysms[4,5] are a rare cause of fourth nerve palsy and we do not routinely recommend cerebral angiography for isolated fourth nerve palsies.

Anterior communicating artery aneurysms (answer choice A) can rarely compress the optic nerve or optic chiasm and present with visual loss in one or both eyes. Aneurysms of the posterior communicating artery (answer choice B) are more commonly associated with an ipsilateral, typically pupil-involved, third nerve palsy. Aneurysms of the vertebral artery (answer choice D) can rarely cause lower cranial nerve deficits that do not normally affect ocular motility. Vertebral artery dissection and pseudoaneurysm formation, however, could produce brainstem ischemia and skew deviation that could mimic a fourth nerve palsy.

The solution to Question 2 is D.

The typical presenting symptom in patients with unilateral fourth nerve palsy is binocular vertical diplopia that is often accompanied by a compensatory contralateral, rather than ipsilateral (answer choice A), head tilt.[1] The head tilt minimizes the vertical diplopia by moving the eye away from the paretic superior oblique's field of action. Rarely, however, some patients with fourth nerve palsy may adopt an ipsilateral rather than contralateral head tilt to cause an increase in the vertical deviation, which produces a greater distance between the two images and an increased ability for some patients to ignore the second image. The superior oblique muscle, which is innervated by the fourth cranial nerve, has three functions that are dependent on the position of gaze: (1) primary function: incyclotorsion (or intorsion) of the eye; (2) secondary function: depression (or infraduction) of the globe when the eye is in the adducted position; and (3) tertiary function: abduction of the eye in downgaze.[2,6] The direct antagonist of the superior oblique muscle is the ipsilateral inferior oblique muscle. With a fourth nerve palsy, there is *underaction* of the ipsilateral superior oblique muscle and thus apparent *overaction* of the now unopposed ipsilateral inferior oblique muscle, which acts (among other functions) to elevate the eye. Therefore, a hypertropia will be observed in the affected eye which is greater in contralateral gaze (due to overaction of the ipsilateral inferior oblique in adduction) and greater in head tilt towards the affected eye.

Hypotropia of the affected eye and hypertropia of the unaffected eye are suggestive of other extraocular muscle deficits (e.g., skew deviation, thyroid eye disease, and myasthenia gravis). Excyclotorsion of the affected eye is typically seen in fourth nerve palsy. Hypoglobus describes an inferiorly displaced globe within the orbit, which can typically be the result of trauma or an orbital lesion.

The solution to Question 3 is C.

Excyclotorsion of the affected eye, due to weakness of the incyclotorsion action of the superior oblique muscle, can produce symptoms in a patient with a fourth nerve palsy. The torsion can be seen subjectively, can be a barrier to fusion, and can be observed objectively on the dilated fundus exam (see Fig. 11.2). The torsion can also be measured subjectively using a double Maddox rod.[7] The patient reports the subjective tilt in the two lines while wearing the double Maddox rods over each eye in a trial frame. These two lines (one from each eye) are

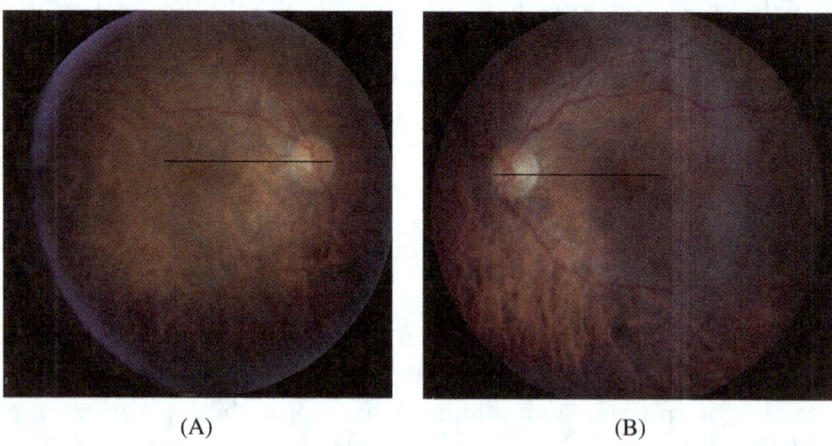

(A)   (B)

Fig. 11.2.   The right eye (A) shows a small degree of excyclodeviation, evident from the straight line drawn from the fovea extending through the optic disc, demonstrating that the fovea is more than one third of a disc diameter below the center of the optic disc. In the left eye (B), no torsion is present, demonstrated by the straight line drawn through the center of the optic disc, showing the fovea is located approximately one third of a disc diameter below the center of the optic disc.

normally viewed as parallel (perpendicular to the orientation of the two vertical Maddox rods), but in patients with torsion, one or both eyes show tilt in the viewed horizontal lines. The patient can rotate the lenses in the trial frame and the amount of torsion can be directly measured. Anatomically, the fovea is located about one third of a disc diameter below the center of the optic disc (see Fig. 11.2B). If the fovea is lower than expected, then excyclotorsion is present. The Hirschberg test (answer choice A), the cover-uncover test (answer choice B), and single Maddox rod (answer choice D) are not as useful in detecting cyclodeviations as either the double Maddox rod test or objective documentation of torsion on fundoscopic exam.

The solution to Question 4 is D.

Bilateral cranial nerve four palsies account for up to 10–30% of all fourth nerve palsy cases.[8–10] Bilateral palsies are typically the result of trauma, but can also be caused by increased intracranial pressure, Chiari I malformation, midbrain tumor, stroke, or other patholo-gies.[11–13] In primary gaze, there is often minimal or no ocular misalignment (the vertical deviation in each eye balances out the primary position deviation) due to the bilateral nature of involved vertically acting muscles (answer choice A). Decreased superior oblique muscle function can produce an esotropia that is worse in downgaze due to the weakened tertiary abducting action of the supe-rior oblique muscle. This produces a V-pattern esotropia (not exotropia, as stated in answer choice C) when there is a 15-prism-diopter or greater difference between upgaze and downgaze.[2] In bilateral superior oblique palsy, the hypertropia will alternate so that the hypertropic eye is contralateral (not ipsilateral) to the direction of gaze and ipsilateral to the direction of head tilt[2,7] (answer choice B). In bilateral cranial nerve four palsies, there is often a large angle of excyclotorsion (> 10 degrees) that is accompanied by prominent tor-sional diplopia. Thus, in any patient with excyclotorsion greater than 10 degrees, bilateral superior oblique palsy should be suspected (answer choice D). Unilateral, isolated fourth nerve palsy can usually be attributed to traumatic, ischemic, or congenital palsy. Unexplained, bilateral, non-traumatic fourth nerve palsies should undergo imaging with attention to the dorsal midbrain.

The solution to Question 5 is A.

The initial evaluation of any patient presenting with a unilateral vertical misalignment involves using the Parks–Bielschowsky three-step test to determine the paretic muscle.[1] Only eight muscles are involved in vertical ocular alignment: the right superior rectus (RSR), the right inferior rectus (RIR), the right superior oblique (RSO), the right inferior oblique (RIO), the left superior rectus (LSR), the left inferior rectus (LIR), the left superior oblique (LSO), and the left inferior oblique (LIO). Each of the three steps of the Parks–Bielschowsky test is designed to eliminate one or more of the muscles listed above such that after all three steps are performed, only one muscle is isolated as the affected, or paretic muscle.

The first step of the test involves determining the hypertropic eye. If there is a right hypertropia (RHT), the paretic muscle can be either of the right eye depressors (RIR, RSO) or either of the left eye elevators (LSR, LIO). Conversely, in the case of left hypertropia, the paretic muscle can be the LIR or LSO, or RSR, or RIO.

The second step involves determining whether the hypertropia is worse in right or left gaze. The recti muscles have a greater vertical action when the eye is in an abducted position, while the oblique muscles have a greater vertical action when the eye is in an adducted position. Thus, for the affected or hypertropic eye, the paretic muscle must be a vertical rectus muscle if the hypertropia worsens in abduction, or an oblique muscle if the hypertropia worsens in adduction. For example, for a right hypertropia, if the RHT worsens in right gaze, the paretic muscle is the RIR or LIO. If the right hypertropia worsens in left gaze, the paretic muscle is the RSO or LSR.

The third step is to determine whether the hypertropia is worse on right or left head tilt. The superior muscles (SR, SO) intort the eye, while the inferior muscles (IR, IO) extort the eye. In a head tilt, the eye ipsilateral to the direction of the tilt (i.e., right eye in right head tilt or left eye in left head tilt) will intort (through action of the SR and

SO), and the contralateral eye will extort (through action of the IO and IR). Thus, the hypertropia, or vertical deviation, will be increased in a head tilt ipsilateral to the affected eye if one of the intorting muscles is paretic (SR or SO). Likewise, the hypertropia will be increased in a head tilt contralateral to the affected eye if one of the extorting muscles is paretic (IR or IO).

Thus, after the conclusion of the three steps, only one muscle should remain as the affected, or paretic muscle, through the process of elimination. An additional fourth step can be added to test for the presence of any torsion using the double Maddox rod. In the case of a right fourth nerve palsy, the RHT should be worse in left gaze and right head tilt with excyclotorsion OD. A left hypertropia (i.e., a right hypotropia) would not be expected in a right fourth nerve palsy.

The solution to Question 6 is C.

In most series, the most common cause of acute, isolated fourth nerve palsy is head trauma, accounting for up to 40% of all cases.[8–10] The fourth cranial nerve exits dorsally, is crossed, and is the longest of all the cranial nerves. The fourth nerve is thus most susceptible to shearing injury at the free margin of the tentorium cerebelli and traumatic cases are often bilateral. In cases of traumatic fourth nerve palsy, the diplopia will often have a clear temporal relationship to the previous head trauma and may improve or remain static after onset. Unfortunately, some patients do not recall the traumatic event or have only minor trauma as the inciting cause.

Microvascular ischemia can also cause an isolated fourth nerve palsy, particularly in individuals with multiple vasculopathic risk factors such as diabetes mellitus.[11] Non-vasculopathic causes of isolated trochlear nerve palsy are rare, but can include clinical entities such as a lacunar midbrain infarction (answer choice B), subarachnoid hemorrhage, or posterior fossa tumor. However, these etiologies are typically associated with other neurological and clinical findings ("defined by the company it keeps").[12–15] Patients above the age of 50 years should undergo evaluation for giant cell arteritis (GCA), a type of systemic vasculitis (answer choice D), as clinically indicated, but fourth nerve palsy would be an unusual finding in GCA. Nevertheless, elderly patients should be queried regarding associated typical signs and symptoms (i.e., scalp tenderness, jaw claudication, temporal nodularity, or acute visual loss) for GCA. Myasthenia gravis (answer choice A) should be also in the differential diagnosis of any pupil-sparing, painless ophthalmoplegia and can mimic a fourth nerve palsy but is an uncommon cause. If, however, the patient has variability or fatigue, other signs of myasthenia gravis (e.g., ptosis, other ocular or systemic signs), or has a three-step test that implicates an unusual muscle (e.g., inferior oblique), then evaluation should proceed for myasthenia gravis.

The solution to Question 7 is B.

Congenital fourth nerve palsy is a common etiology in patients with isolated fourth nerve palsy.[15] The symptoms and signs may be subtle or compensated for in childhood and may only worsen in adulthood due to decompensation (thought to be a breakdown of vertical fusion rather than progressive superior oblique dysfunction). This type of patient often complains of neck pain from chronic head tilting and torticollis or may have facial asymmetry or sternocleidomastoid hypertrophy. Old photographs of the patient showing a longstanding head tilt will often help in establishing the congenital nature of the diagnosis and large vertical fusional amplitudes (greater than 6–8-prism-diopters) in primary gaze are also more suggestive of congenital cases.[1,2] Excyclotorsion is usually asymptomatic in congenital cases but is more likely symptomatic in acquired cases.

Causes of increased intracranial pressure (answer choice A), particularly idiopathic intracranial hypertension (IIH), are important considerations, especially in obese female patients of childbearing age.[13] However, elevated intracranial pressure is more commonly associated with a non-localizing sixth nerve palsy than a fourth nerve palsy. Although inflammatory, neoplastic, and infectious etiologies (answer choices C and D) can be rare causes of fourth nerve palsy, they would not be typical etiologies.[16]

The solution to Question 8 is C.

The initial step in any fourth nerve palsy case involves determining whether the cranial nerve deficit is isolated or non-isolated (i.e., are other neurological signs and symptoms present?).[2] If the fourth nerve palsy is non-isolated, neuroimaging is typically indicated and should be directed at the anatomical location of neurological pathology. Important etiologies of non-isolated fourth nerve palsies can include intracranial malignancy, intracranial hemorrhage, infarction, demyelinating disease, myasthenia gravis, cavernous sinus thrombosis, orbital apex syndrome, and toxic/nutritional polyneuropathy.[17–20] In patients with an isolated fourth nerve palsy, it is important to first consider the more common congenital and traumatic etiologies. Patients with vasculopathic trochlear nerve palsy should not have progression or worsening of their symptoms, which should improve or resolve within three to six months.[21]

If symptoms do not improve or progress, the initial diagnosis should be questioned and the patient should undergo neuroimaging, preferably MRI of the brain and orbits with and without contrast and fat suppression.[22] It is also important to re-evaluate for syndromes that can initially mimic a fourth nerve palsy such as myasthenia gravis, giant cell arteritis (in an older patient), skew deviation, and thyroid eye disease. Oral steroids (answer choice A) can be given for a variety of inflammatory etiologies but would be an inappropriate next step in a patient without a clearly defined disease process. B-scan ultrasound (answer choice B) can accurately image intraocular structures and give valuable information on the status of the lens, vitreous, retina, choroid, and sclera. Thus, combined A- and B-scan ultrasonography can be helpful in the evaluation for thyroid eye disease (looking for enlarged extraocular muscles) but neuroimaging is still superior in the evaluation of a worsening fourth nerve palsy. Strabismus surgery (answer choice D), usually consisting of inferior oblique weakening (myomectomy with disinsertion, recession, etc.) or less commonly a superior oblique strengthening procedure, is considered only after conservative measures fail, an etiologic diagnosis has been established, and there has been stability of the ocular misalignment for a period of at least six months. A trial of base-down prism over the hypertropic eye is usually attempted prior to surgery; however, this method does not correct torsional diplopia and many patients find prism correction unsatisfactory if they have a large torsional component as the barrier to fusion.

SUMMARY

A unilateral fourth nerve palsy typically presents with binocular vertical diplopia, a compensatory contralateral head tilt, and excyclotorsion of the affected eye. On examination, the affected eye will have a hypertropia that is larger in contralateral gaze and ipsilateral head tilt (i.e., the three-step test). Common etiologies of fourth nerve palsy include head trauma, congenital, and microvascular ischemia. Other important but less common etiologies include lacunar midbrain infarction, subarachnoid hemorrhage, giant cell arteritis, demyelinating disease, myasthenia gravis, and posterior fossa tumors. Bilateral fourth nerve palsy has a unique presentation characterized by minimal ocular misalignment in primary gaze, an alternating hypertropia (contralateral to the direction of gaze) and ipsilateral to the direction of head tilt, and an esotropia in either eye that is worse in downgaze (classified as a V-pattern esotropia if there is at least a 15-prism-diopter difference between upgaze and downgaze), and greater, bilateral excyclotorsion. Bilateral fourth nerve palsy is most often due to head trauma but can also result from other intracranial pathologies.

When evaluating a patient with a fourth nerve palsy, it is important to first establish whether the cranial nerve deficit is isolated or non-isolated. Non-isolated cases require further neuroimaging, preferably magnetic resonance imaging of the brain and orbits with and without contrast and fat suppression. Isolated fourth nerve palsy with a clear traumatic, congenital, or microvascular cause typically does not require further diagnostic workup and normally resolves within three to six months. If the deficit fails to improve or progresses within this time interval, neuroimaging is recommended and the patient should be re-evaluated for systemic diseases that can initially mimic a fourth nerve palsy such as myasthenia gravis, giant cell arteritis, skew deviation, and thyroid eye disease.

REFERENCES

1. Lee AG, Brazis PW. (2003) *Clinical Pathways in Neuro-Ophthalmology: An Evidence-Based Approach*, 2nd ed. Thieme Medical Publishing, New York, NY.
2. Brazis PW. (2009) Isolated palsies of cranial nerves III, IV, and VI. *Semin Neurology* **29**:14–28.
3. Miller NR. (1996) The ocular motor nerves. *Curr Opin Neurol* **9**:21–25.
4. Agostinis C, Caverni L, Moschini L, *et al.* (1992) Paralysis of fourth cranial nerve due to superior-cerebellar artery aneurysm. *Neurology* **42**:457–458.
5. Collins TE, Mehalic TF, White TK, Pezzuti RT. (1992) Trochlear nerve palsy as the sole initial sign of an aneurysm of the superior cerebellar artery. *Neurosurgery* **30**:258–261.
6. Hamilton SR. (1999) Neuro-ophthalmology of eye movement disorders. *Curr Opin Ophthalmol* **10**:405–410.
7. Biernacki R. (2011) Evaluation techniques for paretic vertical strabismus. *Am Orthopt J* **61**:2–5.
8. Baker RS, Epstein AD. (1991) Ocular motor abnormalities from head trauma. *Surv Ophthalmol* **35**:245–267.
9. Mollan SP, Edwards JH, Price A, *et al.* (2009) Aetiology and outcomes of adult superior oblique palsies: a modern series. *Eye (Lond)* **23**:640–644.
10. Keane JR. (1993) Fourth nerve palsy: historical review and study of 215 patients. *Neurology* **43**:2439–2443.
11. Jacobson DM, McCanna TD, Layde PM. (1994) Risk factors for ischemic ocular motor nerve palsies. *Arch Ophthalmol* **112**:961–966.
12. Simon S, Sandhu A, Selva D, Crompton JL. (2009) Bilateral trochlear nerve palsies following dorsal midbrain haemorrhage. *N Z Med J* **122**:72–75.
13. Mielke C, Alexander MS, Anand N. (2001) Isolated bilateral trochlear nerve palsy as the first clinical sign of a metastatic [correction of metastasic] bronchial carcinoma. *Am J Ophthalmol* **132**:593–594.
14. Patton N, Beatty S, Lloyd IC. (2000) Bilateral sixth and fourth cranial nerve palsies in idiopathic intracranial hypertension. *J R Soc Med* **93**:80–81.
15. Von Noorden GK, Murray E, Wong SY. (1986) Superior oblique paralysis. A review of 270 cases. *Arch Ophthalmol* **104**:1771–1776.
16. Mansour AM, Reinecke RD. (1986) Central trochlear palsy. *Surv Ophthalmol* **5**:279–297.
17. Rucker CW. (1996) The causes of paralysis of the third, fourth and sixth cranial nerves. *Am J Ophthalmol* **61**:353–358.
18. Richards BW, Jones FR, Younge BR. (1992) Causes and prognosis in 4278 cases of paralysis of the oculomotor, trochlear and abducens cranial nerves. *Am J Ophthalmol* **113**:489–496.

19. Kline LB. (1995) Cavernous sinus/orbital apex syndrome. In: Tusa RJ, Newman SA (eds), *Neuro-ophthalmological Disorders.* Marcel Dekker, New York, NY, pp. 291–298.

20. Godani M, Giorli E, Traverso E, *et al.* (2013) Ramsay Hunt syndrome with trochlear nerve involvement and EEG abnormalities: multicranial neuritis or encephalitis? *J Clin Virol* **56**:277–279.

21. Fujioka T, Segawa F, Ogawa K, *et al.* (1995) Ischemic and hemorrhagic brain stem lesions mimicking diabetic ophthalmoplegia. *Clin Neurol Neurosurg* **97**:167–171.

22. Murchison AP, Gilbert ME, Savino PJ. (2011) Neuroimaging and acute ocular motor mononeuropathies: a prospective study. *Arch Ophthalmol* **129**:301–305.

12

Sixth Nerve Palsy

Nagham Al-Zubidi MD, Rabeea Khan BS,
Arielle Spitze MD, Sushma Yalamanchili MD,
and Andrew G. Lee MD

CASE

A 62-year-old male presented with an acute onset of painless horizontal and vertical binocular diplopia of three weeks' duration. He had no symptoms of giant cell arteritis or myasthenia gravis. Past surgical history was significant for knee reconstructive surgery. He was allergic to penicillin. His family history was significant for stroke and hypertension. His social history was significant for a 54-pack-year smoking history.

On examination, his best-corrected visual acuity was 20/20 bilaterally (OU). Color vision was 14/14 Ishihara color plates OU. Pupils were 4 mm in the dark and 2 mm in the light and there was no relative afferent pupillary defect (RAPD). Extraocular motility showed a mild abduction deficit in the left eye (OS), and an esotropia (ET) of 4 prism-diopters (PD) in primary position and 20 ET on left gaze but he was straight in right gaze. Intraocular pressure, slit lamp, and funduscopic examinations were normal OU.

Question 1	Question 2
Which of the following is the most likely cause of acute isolated sixth nerve palsy in adults over the age of 50 years?	**Which of the following is the most likely presenting symptom of an isolated, right sixth nerve palsy?**
A. Meningioma **B.** Microvascular ischemia **C.** Giant cell arteritis **D.** Intracranial hypertension	**A.** Binocular vertical diplopia, worse on right gaze **B.** Monocular horizontal diplopia, worse on right gaze **C.** Binocular horizontal diplopia, worse on right gaze **D.** Binocular horizontal diplopia, worse on left gaze
Question 3	Question 4
Which of the following signs suggests the diagnosis of thyroid eye disease over isolated sixth nerve palsy?	**Which of the following findings would be most likely to be present in a patient with a non-localizing sixth nerve palsy due to idiopathic intracranial hypertension?**
A. Positive forced duction testing **B.** Incomitant esotropia **C.** Ipsilateral abduction deficit **D.** Deviation worse in the direction of the presumed paretic lateral rectus	**A.** Papilledema bilaterally **B.** Ipsilateral or contralateral ptosis **C.** Bitemporal hemianopsia **D.** Relative afferent pupillary defect
Question 5	Question 6
Which of the following signs would be most suggestive that myasthenia gravis was the cause of a presumed sixth nerve palsy?	**Which of the following radiographic signs is most consistent with thyroid eye disease (TED) as the etiology for an esotropia?**
A. Lid retraction and lid lag **B.** Proptosis and lid retraction **C.** Diplopia and proptosis **D.** Variability and fatigue	**A.** Atrophy of the lateral rectus muscle without involvement of the tendon **B.** Enlargement of the superior ophthalmic vein and extraocular muscles **C.** Enlargement of extraocular muscles without involvement of the tendons **D.** Enlargement of extraocular muscles with involvement of the tendons

Question 7	Question 8
Which of the following is the most likely localization for an isolated sixth nerve palsy?	Which of the following radiographic modalities is the best initial study for an acute, non-traumatic, neurologically isolated sixth cranial nerve palsy in a healthy 20-year-old man?
A. Medulla **B.** Pons **C.** Midbrain **D.** Thalamus	**A.** B-scan ultrasound of the orbit **B.** Computed tomography (CT) scan of the orbit with contrast **C.** CT angiography (CTA) **D.** Magnetic resonance imaging (MRI) of the head with contrast
Question 9	**Question 10**
Which of the following is the best first-line treatment for a comitant, small-angle cranial nerve six palsy?	Which of the following is the most likely prognosis of an isolated, vasculopathic cranial nerve VI palsy?
A. Correcting base-out prisms **B.** Botulinum toxin injection **C.** Medial rectus resection **D.** Medial rectus disinsertion	**A.** Approximately two thirds resolve spontaneously within three months **B.** Approximately half resolve spontaneously within three days **C.** Approximately two thirds experience recurrence **D.** Lack of recovery

EXPLANATIONS

The solution to Question 1 is B.

Sixth nerve palsy is the most common ocular motor palsy, and representing 40–50% of the total in most series.[1,2] Population studies had shown that in adults over the age of 50 years, the leading cause of sixth nerve palsy is microvascular ischemia.[1] In contrast, neoplasm is a leading cause of sixth nerve palsy in children.[1,2] Despite modern neuroimaging techniques, approximately 20–30% of cases remain of unknown etiology (i.e., idiopathic sixth nerve palsy).[2] Giant cell arteritis and intracranial hypertension are other important but less common etiologies for sixth nerve palsy.[2] Other signs and symptoms of giant cell arteritis (e.g., headache, jaw pain, visual loss) should be sought in elderly patients with sixth nerve palsy and other signs of increased intracranial pressure (e.g., papilledema, headache) should be noted in any patient of any age with a non-localizing sixth nerve palsy. An erythrocyte sedimentation rate (ESR) and C-reactive protein (CRP) could be considered even in presumed vasculopathic ocular motor cranial neuropathy but the yield would be low in an otherwise asymptomatic 50-year-old patient. The clinician should ensure that the sixth nerve palsy is isolated before making the diagnosis of vasculopathic sixth nerve palsy. An alternative diagnosis should be suspected if the sixth nerve palsy is non-isolated, if there is progression, emergence of new symptoms or signs or lack of improvement. In addition, some authors believe that neuroimaging should be performed even in unilateral, acute, neurologically isolated, and presumed ischemic ocular motor cranial neuropathy because of the small percentage of intracranial etiologies mimicking an ischemic palsy. Meningioma especially involving the skull base, clivus, cerebellopontine angle, or cavernous sinus could produce an isolated sixth nerve palsy but would not be expected to be acute. Nevertheless, progressive palsies or those that do not improve should be considered for neuroimaging to exclude a compressive etiology.

The solution to Question 2 is C.

Isolated sixth nerve palsy results in impairment of the ipsilateral lateral rectus muscle, which is responsible for abduction of the eye. As a result, the medial rectus muscle is unopposed and an incomitant esotropia develops. The ocular deviation and therefore typically the symptoms of diplopia are thus worse in ipsilateral gaze. Over time however the esotropia may become more comitant (equal in all gaze positions). In all patients presenting with diplopia, it is important to assess whether the diplopia is monocular or binocular. With a sixth nerve palsy, the patient experiences binocular horizontal diplopia that is worse with gaze in the direction of the impaired lateral rectus

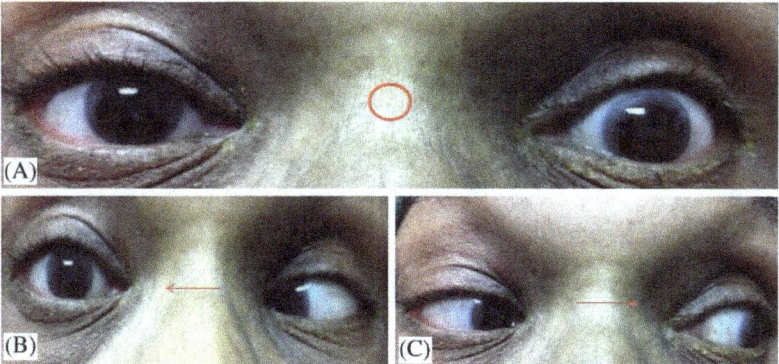

Fig. 12.1. Motility figure in a sixth nerve palsy. (A) On primary gaze, there is esotropia of the right eye. (B) Impaired abduction of the right eye on attempted right gaze. (C) Intact adduction of the right eye and intact abduction of the left eye on attempted left gaze.

muscle as the disparity of eye movement is most pronounced in the direction of action of the paretic muscle (as shown in Fig. 12.1).[2]

In general, monocular diplopia implies an optical problem in the affected eye or eyes (bilateral but monocular diplopia). Although a small vertical deviation (less than 2–4 prism-diopters) can occur in isolated sixth nerve palsy, most patients complain of binocular horizontal diplopia only. Any vertical deviation greater than a few prism diopters should be considered suspicious for an additional or alternative diagnosis (e.g., concomitant skew deviation, third or fourth nerve palsy, thyroid eye disease, or myasthenia gravis).

The solution to Question 3 is A.

In thyroid eye disease a restrictive myopathy (rather than a paretic process) can produce an incomitant esotropia, an ipsilateral abduction deficit, and a deviation worse in the direction of the presumed paretic lateral rectus muscle that can mimic the presentation of a sixth nerve palsy. TED is due to an inflammatory enlargement and secondary fibrotic contraction of the extraocular muscles.[1] Although the inferior rectus is the most commonly affected muscle (resulting in restriction on upgaze), the medial rectus is the second most affected, and can present with abduction deficit and an incomitant ET.[1] However, restrictive myopathy like TED can be differentiated from an acute isolated paretic sixth nerve palsy with positive forced duction testing.[1–3] Lid retraction, lid lag, and proptosis are other common signs of TED that would not be expected in an isolated sixth nerve palsy but may be variably present with TED. Thus, TED should be in the differential diagnosis of any patient with a presumed sixth nerve palsy.

The solution to Question 4 is A.

An isolated sixth nerve palsy can be a non-localizing sign of increased intracranial pressure (ICP). In idiopathic intracranial hypertension (IIH) (also known as pseudotumor cerebri), a sixth nerve palsy is a common cause of binocular horizontal diplopia and occurs in up to one fourth of cases of IIH.[4] Other associated signs and symptoms of increased ICP may include papilledema (see Fig. 12.2), headache, and transient visual obscurations.

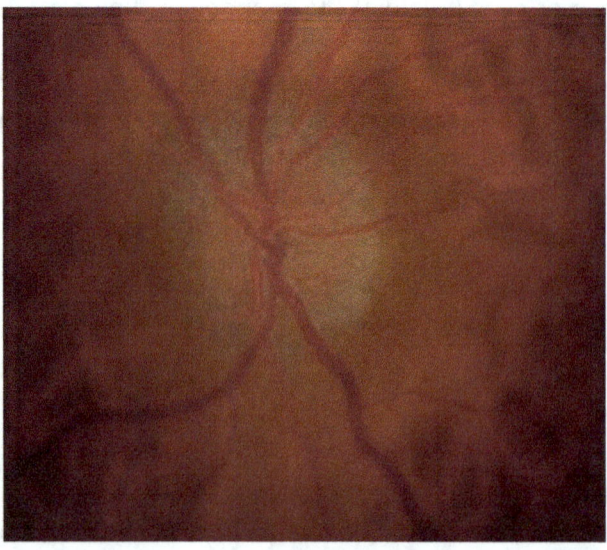

Fig. 12.2. Fundus photo showing papilledema (a sign of increased intracranial pressure).

Normal or even slit-like ventricles are seen on neuroimaging in IIH, and elevated opening pressure on lumbar puncture with normal cerebrospinal fluid content in the setting of normal neuroimaging is diagnostic in cases of IIH presenting with cranial nerve VI palsy. Unfortunately, although papilledema is often present in these cases of IIH, it may be absent too.[4] Bitemporal hemianopsia is a visual field defect that localizes to the optic chiasm and would not be expected in IIH where enlargement of the blind spot and nerve fiber layer–type visual field defects are more common. An RAPD can be seen in asymmetric or unilateral papilledema cases in IIH but is atypical. Thus every patient with a sixth nerve palsy should have evaluation for papilledema which might suggest that the sixth nerve palsy is due to increased intracranial pressure including IIH.

The solution to Question 5 is D.

Myasthenia gravis can produce any pattern of pupil-sparing, non-proptotic ophthalmoplegia and can mimic a unilateral or bilateral sixth nerve palsy. Weakness that is variable and worsens with muscle use (i.e., fatigue) that is variable in duration, severity, or laterality is suggestive of myasthenia gravis.[1,5] Ptosis (rather than lid retraction seen in TED) is a common presenting sign of myasthenia gravis and is likewise variable and exacerbated by fatigue. Ptosis would not be expected in an isolated sixth nerve palsy. Lid retraction, lid lag, and proptosis are common signs of TED which can interestingly occur in combination with myasthenia gravis as both conditions are autoimmune in origin. Diplopia however is a non-specific complaint and would occur in neurogenic, myogenic, and neuromuscular junction etiologies. Every patient who has a presumed sixth nerve palsy should be queried and examined for symptoms or signs of myasthenia gravis.

The solution to Question 6 is C.

TED produces a restrictive myopathy that can mimic esotropia and abduction deficit of a sixth nerve palsy. TED usually results

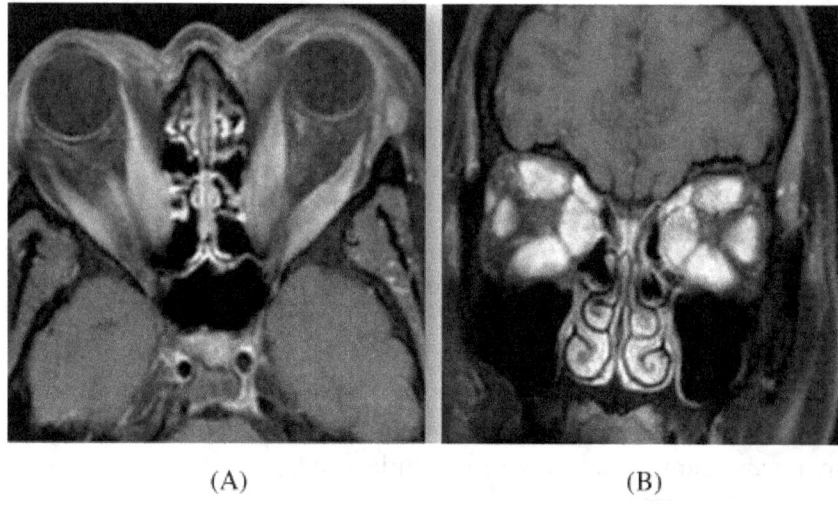

(A)   (B)

Fig. 12.3. MRI T1-weighted with fat suppression and contrast: axial (A) and coronal (B) showing extraocular muscle enlargement and tendon sparing consistent with thyroid eye disease.

radiographically in bilateral symmetric enlargement of multiple extraocular muscles that can be seen on CT, MR, or ultrasound of the orbit. This distinctive radiographic sign is seen for example in the orbital T1 post-contrast MRI (see Fig. 12.3).[1,3] The order of extraocular muscle involvement in TED is typically inferior rectus > medial rectus > superior rectus > lateral rectus muscle. Classically, the tendon in TED is spared as opposed to orbital inflammatory pseudotumor, but there are exceptions. Enlargement of the superior ophthalmic vein is the distinctive radiographic sign of carotid-cavernous fistula (CCF) although the CCF can also produce extraocular muscle enlargement. Atrophy of the lateral rectus muscle is seen in denervation atrophy and can be a sign of chronic and longstanding sixth nerve palsy. Thus, in patients suspected of having TED as the cause for an esotropia, imaging might be necessary and should include the orbit to look for medial rectus muscle enlargement and sparing of the tendon.

The solution to Question 7 is B.

All of the ocular motor cranial nerve nuclei originate in the brainstem. The midbrain contains the nuclei and fascicles for cranial nerves III and IV. The pons contains nuclei for cranial nerves VI, VII, and VIII.[6] The cranial nerve VI nucleus is located in the dorsal caudal pons and exits the brainstem at the pontomedullary junction.[1] The facial nerve is often concurrently damaged in this dorsal pontine location because of its close proximity to the cranial nerve VI nucleus.[1] The medulla contains the lower cranial nerves, including IX, X, XI, and XII, but not VI.[6] Thalamic lesions can produce supranuclear ocular deviations (including thalamic esotropia) and skew deviation. A lesion in any part of the brain or brainstem might produce increased intracranial pressure-related sixth nerve palsy as a non-localizing finding but only pontine lesions can produce a fascicular sixth nerve palsy. The sixth nerve nucleus however is the final common pathway for horizontal gaze and therefore nuclear sixth nerve lesions produce a horizontal gaze palsy and not the ispilateral abduction deficit and incomitant ET seen in sixth nerve palsy.

The solution to Question 8 is D.

The evaluation for an isolated and presumed vasculopathic sixth nerve palsy is controversial but many sources suggest that watchful waiting for improvement is appropriate for up to two to three months when vasculopathic risk factors are present. In a 20-year-old non-vasculopathic patient, neuroimaging would be recommended even for an isolated palsy. Consideration for TED and myasthenia gravis should be made clinically. Neuroimaging (preferably contrast-enhanced MRI following the course of the sixth nerve) is indicated if the sixth nerve palsy is not neurologically isolated, is progressive, or if the presumed vasculopathic sixth nerve palsy worsens or fails to improve after initial observation. An emergent head CT may be preferred over MRI in some settings (e.g., the emergency room) especially when there is a history of trauma, bone, bleeding, or foreign body evaluation or a faster scan is required. However, in non-traumatic cases where there is a neurologically isolated sixth cranial nerve palsy, MRI of the head with and without contrast following the course of the sixth nerve is the imaging modality of choice if there is no contraindication.[1,7]

Although orbital ultrasound, CT without contrast of the orbit, or MRI of the orbit can detect enlargement of extraocular muscles and may be useful for evaluating thyroid-related ophthalmopathy mimicking a sixth nerve palsy, they would not be considered the best initial imaging study for evaluating the course of the sixth cranial nerve anatomy intracranially. CT angiography is useful for excluding intracranial aneurysms as in third nerve palsy but is less useful for sixth nerve palsy where aneurysm is less of a diagnostic consideration.

The solution to Question 9 is A.

Correcting prisms or patching are first-line symptomatic treatment for diplopia as they are non-invasive and reversible options.[1,8] Botulinum toxin injection is a reasonable temporizing measure, especially for traumatic sixth nerve palsy, as relaxing the medial rectus allows the lateral rectus to better recover function.[9] Strabismus surgery is generally reserved for patients who fail or are intolerant to patching or initial prism therapy and who have stable ocular deviations.

The solution to Question 10 is A.

The majority of idiopathic sixth cranial nerve palsies resolve within three months and vasculopathic sixth nerve palsy also typically resolves (up to 86% of cases). Sixth nerve palsy, however, depending on the etiology, may recur in up to one third of patients and these patients may require repeat diagnostic evaluations.[1,8] Patients with recurrence, progression, bilateral involvement, or lack of recovery should probably undergo further evaluation including neuroimaging (preferably contrast MRI following the course of the sixth nerve) and consideration for additional laboratory studies (e.g., thyroid and myasthenia gravis) or lumbar puncture (e.g., increased intracranial pressure, meningeal disease). Rapid spontaneous recovery (less than three weeks) can also be seen in myasthenia gravis or in other mimics of sixth nerve palsy (e.g., accommodative spasm). Recurrent isolated vasculopathic sixth nerve palsy is uncommon but has been reported and in diabetics recurrent sequential ocular motor cranial mononeuropathies are not uncommon. Multiple simultaneous or rapidly sequential cranial neuropathies however are atypical and should prompt further evaluation for additional diagnosis.

SUMMARY

In adults over the age of 50 years, the leading cause of an acute, neurologically isolated, sixth nerve palsy is microvascular ischemia, while neoplasm is more common in younger adults and in children. An isolated sixth nerve palsy results in an incomitant esotropia and binocular horizontal diplopia that is worse with gaze in the direction of impaired abduction. In thyroid eye disease, a restrictive myopathy can produce an abduction deficit that can mimic a sixth nerve palsy but can usually be differentiated by associated symptoms and signs of thyroid disease and if necessary with forced duction testing. Orbital imaging in these cases might classically show bilateral, symmetric enlargement of multiple extraocular muscles. Isolated sixth nerve palsy can be a non-localizing sign of increased intracranial pressure and occurs in approximately one fourth of cases of IIH. Therefore, all patients with a sixth nerve palsy should be evaluated for papilledema. Ophthalmoplegia mimicking a sixth nerve palsy is an uncommon presentation of myasthenia gravis. Weakness that increases with muscle use or fatigue is suggestive of myasthenia gravis. Cranial nerve VI is often involved early in cases of intracavernous lesions (e.g., carotid aneurysm) and can present with concurrent Horner syndrome. Isolated sixth nerve palsy can also be the presenting or only sign of a clivus lesion (e.g., chordoma). For presumed vasculopathic sixth nerve palsy, watchful waiting for improvement for up to two to three months is reasonable but neuroimaging should be considered if the sixth nerve palsy is not neurologically isolated, is progressive, or if the condition worsens or fails to improve after initial observation. MRI with contrast following the course of the sixth nerve is the imaging modality of choice. Magnetic resonance venography may be necessary if increased intracranial pressure and possible venous sinus thrombosis are considerations in the differential diagnosis. Patching or correcting prisms are first-line treatment with surgical treatment considered only if the condition is stable and symptomatic. Botulinum toxin injection is a reasonable temporizing measure, especially for post-traumatic palsies, but is generally not required if resolution is expected. The majority of idiopathic or vasculopathic sixth cranial nerve palsies resolve within three months but depending on the etiology may recur in up to one third of patients and thus may require additional evaluation.

REFERENCES

1. Goodwin D. (2006) Differential diagnosis and management of acquired sixth cranial nerve palsy. *Optometry* **77**:534–539.
2. Rucker JC. (2012) Diplopia, third nerve palsies, and sixth nerve palsies. In: Roos KL (eds), *Emergency Neurology*. Springer, New York, NY, pp. 113–132.
3. Gonçalves AC, Gebrim EM, Monteiro ML. (2012) Imaging studies for diagnosing Graves' orbitopathy and dysthyroid optic neuropathy. *Clinics (Sao Paulo)* **67**:1327–1334.
4. Quattrone A, Bono F, Fera F, Lavano A. (2006) Isolated unilateral abducens palsy in idiopathic intracranial hypertension without papilledema. *Eur J Neurol* **13**:670–671.
5. Patel SV, Mutyala S, Leske DA, *et al.* (2004) Incidence, associations, and evaluation of sixth nerve palsy using a population-based method. *Ophthalmology* **111**:369–375.
6. Hendelman W. (2006) *Atlas of Functional Neuroanatomy*. CRC Press, Boca Raton, FL.

7. Lee AG, Johnson MC, Policeni BA, Smoker WR. (2009) Imaging for neuro-ophthalmic and orbital disease — a review. *Clin Experiment Ophthalmol* **37**:30–53.
8. Sanders SK, Kawasaki A, Purvin VA. (2002) Long-term prognosis in patients with vasculopathic sixth nerve palsy. *Am J Ophthalmol* **134**:81–84.
9. Kao LY, Chao AN. (2003) Subtenon injection of botulinum toxin for treatment of traumatic sixth nerve palsy. *J Pediatr Ophthalmol Strabismus* **40**:27–30.

13

Orbital Apex Syndrome

Arielle Spitze MD, James D. Kim MD, Nagham Al-Zubidi MD,
Sushma Yalamanchili MD, and Andrew G. Lee MD

CASE

A 70-year-old woman presented with a one-month history of progressive, painful loss of vision in the right eye (OD), a droopy right upper eyelid, and horizontal binocular diplopia. Past medical history was significant for hypertension, diabetes mellitus type II, and breast cancer (status post-mastectomy and -chemotherapy). Review of systems was significant for nausea, vomiting, and malaise. On examination, visual acuity was light perception OD and 20/25 in the left eye (OS). The right pupil measured 5 mm in the dark and was non-reactive to light or accommodation with a relative afferent pupillary defect (RAPD) OD (by reverse testing). The left pupil measured 4 mm in the dark and 3 mm in the light with no light-near dissociation. Ocular motility revealed complete ophthalmoplegia OD but full extraocular movements OS (Fig. 13.1). Anterior segment examination and intraocular pressure measurements were normal in both eyes (OU). External exam showed complete ptosis OD. Hertel exophthalmometry showed 3mm of proptosis OD (23mm OD compared with 20mm OS). Dilated fundus exam revealed diffuse optic disc pallor OD and a normal fundus OS. Magnetic resonance imaging (MRI) of the brain and orbits with and without contrast showed a dural-based extra-axial lesion located within the sella and extending into the right-sided cavernous sinus, superior orbital fissure, planum sphenoidale, and infundibulum (Fig. 13.2). Trans-sphenoidal biopsy revealed diffuse large B-cell lymphoma. The patient underwent staging and was treated with systemic chemotherapy and radiotherapy.

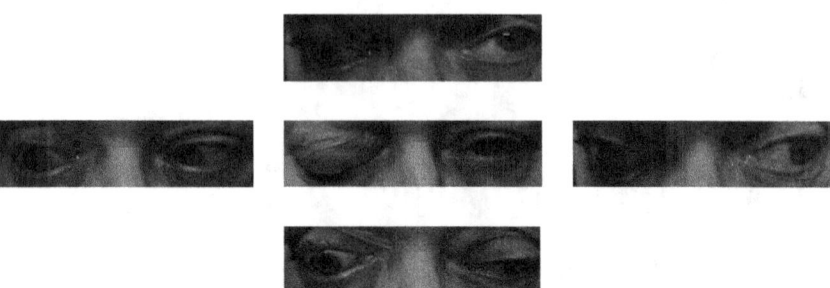

Fig. 13.1. Montage of patient with orbital apex syndrome attempting the cardinal gaze directions. In primary gaze (center picture), there is complete ptosis on the right (cranial nerve III palsy). Note that in all other gaze directions, the right upper lid is being held open by an assistant so that the ocular alignment can be observed. The photos show complete right eye ophthalmoplegia and anisocoria (larger right pupil), implicating the involvement of cranial nerves III, IV and VI. Decreased vision OD and a right RAPD also reveal the additional invlovement of cranial nerve II.

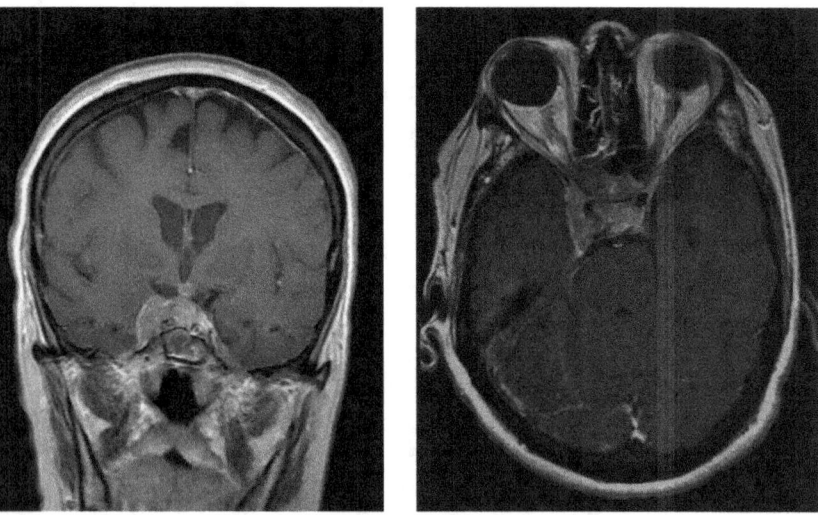

Fig. 13.2. Magnetic resonance imaging of the brain and orbits (both showing T1 images postgadolinium) shows a dural-based extra-axial lesion in the sella, and additionally involving the right cavernous sinus, superior orbital fissure, planum sphenoidale, and infundibulum and extending into the orbital apex, producing the right ophthalmoplegia and concomitant optic neuropathy.

Question 1	Question 2
Which of the following symptoms is most localizing for an orbital apex syndrome?	**Which of the following neoplasms is most likely to be associated with an orbital apex syndrome?**
A. Visual loss and drooping lid **B.** Painful bilateral visual loss **C.** Painless, binocular diplopia **D.** Numbness in the V_3 distribution	**A.** Pituitary adenoma **B.** Glioblastoma multiforme **C.** Meningioma **D.** Craniopharyngioma
Question 3	**Question 4**
Which of the following cranial nerves is most likely to be involved in orbital apex syndrome?	**Which of the following is the best initial imaging for an acute orbital apex syndrome in a diabetic patient in ketoacidosis?**
A. CN III **B.** CN VII **C.** CN VIII **D.** CN V_3	**A.** Non-contrast MRI of the brain **B.** Computed tomography (CT) of the orbit/sinuses **C.** Ultrasound of the orbit **D.** Positron emission tomography (PET)
Question 5	**Question 6**
Which of the following features is most compatible with myasthenia gravis (MG) rather than an orbital apex syndrome?	**Which of the following features best differentiates orbital apex localization from the cavernous sinus?**
A. Anisocoria **B.** Numbness in V_2 **C.** Ipsilateral RAPD **D.** Orbicularis weakness	**A.** Optic neuropathy **B.** Complete ophthalmoplegia **C.** V_1 distribution pain D. Complete ptosis

Question 7	Question 8
Which of the following is the most likely pupil finding in a patient with a left optic neuropathy and a fixed pupil OS due to a left orbital apex syndrome?	**Which of the following indicates an intact fourth nerve function in the presence of an ipsilateral complete third nerve palsy?**
A. OD dilates when light swings OS to OD **B.** OD constricts when light swings from OD to OS **C.** OD dilates when light swings from OD to OS **D.** OS constricts when light swings OS to OD	**A.** Intorsion in downgaze **B.** Extorsion in downgaze **C.** Intorsion in upgaze **D.** Extorsion in upgaze

EXPLANATIONS

The solution to Question 1 is A.

The distinctive symptoms and signs of orbital apex syndrome are ipsilateral visual loss (from an optic neuropathy), binocular diplopia, ptosis, anisocoria, and proptosis.[1] The key clinical signs are the presence of an ipsilateral optic neuropathy and partial or complete ophthalmoplegia that involves multiple cranial nerves or extraocular muscles with or without proptosis.[1] There may be pupil-sparing or pupil involvement with secondary anisocoria and ipsilateral mydriasis (third nerve palsy) or miosis (Horner syndrome or aberrant regeneration of the third cranial nerve). Any or all of the structures that enter the orbit via the superior orbital fissure, optic canal, or inferior orbital fissure can be affected in an ipsilateral orbital apex syndrome, but bilateral involvement is rare. Partial or complete ptosis with or without mydriasis may occur when cranial nerve III is affected, as it innervates the dilator muscle of the pupil and the levator palpebrae muscle of the eyelid.[2] Conversely, Horner syndrome might produce a small (1–2 mm) ptosis or upside-down ptosis from involvement of the sympathetically innervated lid retractors (e.g., Müller muscle).[2] Loss of vision is typically due to the optic nerve (cranial nerve II) being involved, but other mechanisms including corneal exposure or hyperopic shift can also occur. Optic nerve involvement can also manifest as visual field defects, dyschromatopsia, or a RAPD in the affected eye. It is important to be able to perform testing for a RAPD using the reverse method because of the possibility of a concomitant efferent pupillary defect (i.e., the ipsilateral pupil is fixed and dilated from a concomitant third nerve palsy). Diplopia can occur if any of the cranial nerves III, IV, or VI are affected, but some patients do not complain of diplopia because of the complete ptosis acting as an occluder, or visual loss from the ipsilateral optic neuropathy precluding appreciation of the second image. Trigeminal numbness in the V_3 distribution is an ominous sign (numb chin syndrome), because it is often due to an infiltrative neoplasm.[3] However, because the third division of the trigeminal nerve (V_3) exits the skull via the foramen ovale, it does not enter the orbital apex and is therefore not seen in isolated orbital apex syndrome.

The solution to Question 2 is C.

There are a myriad of etiologies that have been documented as the cause of orbital apex syndrome including infectious, inflammatory, infiltrative, and neoplastic disorders. Inflammatory causes include sarcoidosis,[4] systemic lupus erythematosus,[5] eosinophilic granulomatosis with polyangiitis (Churg Strauss syndrome, formerly Wegener's granulomatosis),[5,6] Tolosa–Hunt syndrome,[7] giant cell arteritis,[8] orbital inflammatory pseudotumor,[9] and thyroid orbitopathy. Infectious causes include fungal (most notably, mucormycosis[10] and aspergillosis[11]); bacterial (e.g., *Streptococcus* or *Staphylococcus* species, *Mycobacterium tuberculosis*,[12] and *Treponema pallidum* (syphilis)[13]); and viral (e.g., herpes zoster) disease.[14] The differentiating history that should raise the index of suspicion for infectious etiologies is an acute, often painful orbital apex syndrome in a known immunosuppressed host (e.g., organ transplant survivor on immunosuppression or diabetics, especially those with diabetic ketoacidosis), or patients with presenting or predominant symptoms of adjacent paranasal sinus disease (e.g., fungal or bacterial sinusitis).[10] Neoplastic causes can include, most commonly, meningioma, but also nasopharyngeal carcinoma, adenoid cystic carcinoma, squamous cell carcinoma, neurofibroma, ciliary neurinoma, schwannoma, metastatic malignancies (most commonly lung, breast, renal cell, and melanoma), Burkitt lymphoma, non-Hodgkin lymphoma, and leukemia.[1] Orbital apex neoplasms, in contrast to infectious or inflammatory etiologies, typically present with chronic, progressive, painless unilateral ophthalmoplegia, proptosis, and ipsilateral optic neuropathy. However, metastatic lesions or aggressive infiltrative neoplasms such as systemic lymphoma can present more acutely or subacutely.[15] Vascular causes can include carotid-cavernous aneurysms, carotid-cavernous fistulas, cavernous sinus thromboses, or sickle cell anemia. Mucoceles have also been reported as a cause of orbital apex syndrome and may mimic the presentation of neoplasms.[16] Pituitary adenoma, craniopharyngioma, and glioblastoma multiforme are lesions that would only rarely extend into the orbital apex. Suprasellar lesions, however, could mimic an orbital apex presentation by producing ophthalmoplegia due to concurrent cavernous sinus involvement and optic neuropathy from suprasellar extension of the lesion and compression of the intracranial optic nerve.[17]

The solution to Question 3 is A.

Cranial nerves II (optic nerve), III (oculomotor nerve), IV (trochlear nerve), V_1 (ophthalmic division of the trigeminal nerve), and VI (abducens nerve) are the most likely to be involved in orbital apex syndrome since they enter the orbit via the optic canal (II) or superior orbital fissure (III, IV, V_1, VI).[1] When the optic nerve is not involved, the syndrome is more precisely termed a superior orbital fissure syndrome.[1] Similarly, when the optic nerve is involved and the predominant signs are cranial nerves III, IV, V_1, VI, and V_2 (maxillary division of the trigeminal nerve) then cavernous sinus involvement is more likely because V_2 enters the orbit via the inferior orbital fissure.[1] In contrast, lower cranial nerves (i.e., VII, VIII, IX, X, XI, and XII) do not enter the cavernous sinus or the orbit. Orbicularis oculi weakness, however, might be present in a patient with a pupil-sparing, painless ophthalmoplegia due to myasthenia gravis. MG however would not produce pain, numbness, or paresthesias in the trigeminal distribution or an optic neuropathy.

The solution to Question 4 is B.

An acute orbital apex syndrome in an immunocompromised patient, but especially in the setting of diabetic ketoacidosis, is fungal infection (e.g., mucormycosis) until proven otherwise. Although a high-resolution MRI of the brain and orbits with contrast and fat suppression would provide valuable information on intracranial and intraorbital involvement of neoplastic, inflammatory, and infectious etiologies in a patient with orbital apex syndrome,[16] CT of the orbit is faster and can show sinus and bony anatomy better than MRI. In traumatic orbital apex lesions, CT is definitely superior for visualizing bony fractures and hemorrhage, is the procedure of choice when a foreign body is suspected (especially ferromagnetic material where an MRI would be contraindicated), and is a faster and less expensive imaging modality compared with MRI.[1] Unfortunately, MRI may not show fungal hyphae well, since fungi can be hypointense and mimic the MR appearance of a normal air-filled sinus. CT of the orbit and sinus will typically show sinus disease and orbital extension better than MRI and if surgical intervention (e.g., biopsy for fungal disease) is indicated, the otolaryngologist or orbital surgeon will need to evaluate the orbital bony anatomy to a certain level of detail that cannot be seen as well on MRI.[18] Therefore, in the setting of diabetic ketoacidosis and an orbital apex syndrome, CT scan of orbits and sinuses is the preferred imaging modality of choice to evaluate for the presence of invasive fungal disease. Although the main initial treatment is control of the metabolic diabetic ketoacidosis, CT scan can provide important information in preparation for diagnostic surgical biopsy so that appropriate antifungal therapy can be instituted promptly. If the CT shows no lesion or is non-diagnostic, an MRI of the brain and orbit with fat suppression and gadolinium might still be necessary, as MRI is superior to CT for soft tissue anatomy and cavernous sinus disease.[18] MRI of the brain alone might be negative in patients with orbital disease and failure to order an orbital MRI with fat suppression or gadolinium contrast might reduce the sensitivity of the MRI study to detect disease. Full body PET scanning is not the primary imaging study in patients with an orbital apex syndrome, but might be useful for staging or looking for another site for biopsy in suspected sarcoidosis, lymphoma, or metastatic disease.[19,20]

The solution to Question 5 is D.

MG can mimic any painless, pupil sparing, non-proptotic ophthalmoplegia, including both partial or complete ophthalmoplegic presentations of orbital apex syndrome. MG, however, is a disease of the neuromuscular junction and does not produce: clinical involvement of the pupil (i.e., no RAPD and no anisocoria), pain (especially if pain is trigeminal and suggestive of a structural lesion in the orbital apex, superior orbital fissure, or cavernous sinus), proptosis (unless there is concomitant thyroid eye disease with MG), or visual loss.[21] Although MG is a clinical diagnosis, ancillary clinic testing can support the diagnosis (e.g., edrophonium (Tensilon) or neostigmine (Prostigmin) test, ice, or sleep/rest testing).[21] The ice test is an easily-performed bedside or clinic test which involves placing ice packs on the patient's ptotic eyelids for approximately 1 minute and observing for an improvement or resolution of ptosis.[22] The ice test is believed to work in MG because the cooling effect improves neuromuscular transmission. The ice test has a high sensitivity (up to 80%) for ocular MG, but as with all clinical tests, is not 100% specific.[22] Orbicularis weakness is a commonly encountered finding in MG that would not be expected to be present in an orbital apex lesion.

The solution to Question 6 is A.

The ophthalmologist confronted with a unilateral ophthalmoplegia should test for orbicularis weakness (MG), trigeminal function (V_{1-3}), and look for an ipsilateral optic neuropathy (RAPD, visual field defect, optic disc edema or optic disc pallor). Because the optic nerve travels through the optic canal and not the cavernous sinus, an optic neuropathy would not be expected to occur in an isolated cavernous sinus syndrome.[1] An ipsilateral optic neuropathy (visual loss, RAPD) could therefore help distinguish between cavernous sinus syndrome and orbital apex syndrome, since the optic nerve would likely be involved in an orbital apex syndrome due to its location within the orbital apex. Some cavernous sinus lesions, however, can extend into the suprasellar space or along the skull base to involve the intracranial optic nerve. The most common "sins of omission" are failure to check the function of cranial nerves V and VII in patients with diplopia; failure to check for fourth nerve dysfunction in a patient with a complete third nerve palsy; and failure to measure for proptosis in a patient with ophthalmoplegia. The presence of an additional cranial neuropathy (II, V, VII) in a patient with a presumed ischemic vasculopathic ocular motor cranial neuropathy (e.g., diabetic III, IV, or VI cranial neuropathy) would change the diagnosis from small vessel ischemic disease to a possible structural (cavernous sinus or orbital apex) or other non-ischemic etiology.[23]

The solution to Question 7 is C.

A unilateral, fixed, and dilated pupil in a patient with complete ophthalmoplegia would preclude testing for an RAPD by the routine manner (i.e., looking for dilation upon swinging the light from the contralateral unaffected eye to the affected eye). Instead, the clinician should look for an RAPD by the reverse method. Testing for an RAPD by reverse is performed by first using a dim, indirect light shining from below the unaffected eye (attempting not to stimulate the pupil) for the purpose of visualization of the pupil. Then, a second, bright light is used to swing between the eyes looking for dilation of the unaffected pupil upon swinging from the unaffected pupil to the affected pupil. This reverse RAPD actually occurs every time a unilateral or asymmetric optic neuropathy is present, but it is typically easier to see the dilation in the affected eye rather than relying upon observing the dilation in the contralateral eye (i.e., the reverse RAPD). In the setting of an efferent pupillary defect (i.e., a fixed, dilated pupil), however, testing by the reverse method can document an RAPD even with only one working pupil.[2]

The solution to Question 8 is A.

In the setting of a complete third nerve palsy, incyclotorsion in down-gaze (best seen by watching for torsional movement of a horizontal conjunctival vessel in the nasal interpalpebral fissure zone) should be present if the ipsilateral fourth cranial nerve is intact.[24] A concurrent third and fourth cranial nerve palsy would implicate a structural lesion in the orbital apex or cavernous sinus (depending on the presence of other cranial nerve involvement) and should prompt "neuroimaging." This is a particularly important clinical sign when the differential diagnosis includes a possible ischemic isolated cranial nerve III palsy.

SUMMARY

Orbital apex lesions typically present with ipsilateral visual loss, binocular diplopia, anisocoria, ptosis, and proptosis. The characteristic signs include single or multiple ocular motor cranial neuropathies (III, IV, VI, or any combination) causing ophthalmoplegia, optic neuropathy (visual loss, dyschromatopsia, RAPD, optic disc edema, or atrophy), anisocoria, ptosis, and proptosis. The cranial nerves typically affected are those that pass through the superior orbital fissure (III, IV, V_1, VI) and optic canal (II). A wide range of systemic diseases may cause an orbital apex syndrome, including infectious, neoplastic, infiltrative, vascular, inflammatory, or autoimmune disease. A thorough history and review of systems is crucial to narrow the differential diagnosis. Neuroimaging, preferably magnetic resonance imaging of the brain and orbits with contrast and fat suppression, is the preferred imaging modality in most chronic cases but acute cases might benefit from CT of orbits and sinuses (especially if sinus disease is suspected or in a diabetic, ketoacidotic patient where fungal disease is likely to be present). Treatment is determined by the underlying etiology. In presumed inflammatory cases, corticosteroids should be considered only after ruling out infectious causes. However, the diagnosis of an inflammatory etiology (e.g., Tolosa–Hunt syndrome, orbital inflammatory pseudotumor, optic neuritis, optic perineuritis) should be used with caution in patients who are immunosuppressed (especially those with diabetic ketoacidosis) where fungal disease (mucormycosis or aspergillosis) is more likely. In addition, empiric corticosteroid treatment of presumed inflammatory orbital disease, if the diagnosis is indeed fungal in origin, may worsen the disease process. Careful testing of cranial nerves V and VII as well as testing for a RAPD and reverse RAPD (in patients with concomitant efferent pupillary defects) is mandatory to avoid misdiagnosis of a presumed isolated ischemic ocular motor cranial neuropathy.

REFERENCES

1. Yeh S, Foroozan R. (2004) Orbital apex syndrome. *Curr Opin Ophthalmol* **15**:490–498.
2. Duong DK, Leo MM, Mitchell EL. (2008) Neuro-ophthalmology. *Emerg Med Clin North Am* **26**:137–180, vii.
3. Kim YI, An JY, Lee KS, *et al.* (2011) Numb chin syndrome with concomitant painful ophthalmoplegia leading to a diagnosis of diffuse large B cell lymphoma. *Cancer Res Treat* **43**:134–138.
4. Segal EI, Tang RA, Lee AG, *et al.* (2000) Orbital apex lesion as the presenting manifestation of sarcoidosis. *J Neuroophthalmol* **20**:156–158.
5. Mohsenin A, Huang JJ. (2012) Ocular manifestations of systemic inflammatory diseases. *Conn Med* **76**:533–544.
6. Shunmugam M, Morley AM, Graham E, *et al.* (2011) Primary Wegener's granulomatosis of the orbital apex with initial optic nerve infiltration. *Orbit* **30**:24–26.
7. Mendez JA, Arias CR, Sanchez D, *et al.* (2009) Painful ophthalmoplegia of the left eye in a 19-year-old female, with an emphasis in Tolosa-Hunt Syndrome: a case report. *Cases J* **2**:8271.
8. Islam N, Asaria R, Plant GT, Hykin PC. (2003) Giant cell arteritis mimicking idiopathic orbital inflammatory disease. *Eur J Ophthalmol* **13**:392–394.
9. Eftekhari K, Chikwava KR, Katowitz WR. (2011) Idiopathic orbital inflammation leading to unilateral blindness over a 2-day presentation in a child. *Ophthal Plast Reconstr Surg* **27**:e46–47.

10. Gamaletsou MN, Sipsas NV, Roilides E, Walsh TJ. (2012) Rhino-orbital-cerebral mucormycosis. *Curr Infect Dis Rep* **14**:423–434.

11. Siraj CA, Krishnan J, Nair RR, Girija AS. (2005) Invasive aspergillosis producing painful ophthalmoplegia. *J Assoc Physicians India* **53**:901–902.

12. Hughes EH, Petrushkin H, Sibtain NA, *et al.* (2008) Tuberculous orbital apex syndromes. *Br J Ophthalmol* **92**:1511–1517.

13. Currie JN, Coppeto JR, Lessell S. (1988) Chronic syphilitic meningitis resulting in superior orbital fissure syndrome and posterior fossa gumma. A report of two cases followed for 20 years. *J Clin Neuroophthalmol* **8**:145–159.

14. Kurimoto T, Tonari M, Ishizaki N, *et al.* (2011) Orbital apex syndrome associated with herpes zoster ophthalmicus. *Clin Ophthalmol* **5**:1603–1608.

15. Besada E, Hunter M, Bittner B. (2007) An uncommon presentation of orbital apex syndrome. *Optometry* **78**:339–343.

16. Yoon MK, McCulley TJ. (2010) Orbital disease in neuro-ophthalmology. *Neurol Clin* **28**:679–699.

17. Swartz NG, Savino PJ. (1993) Clinical manifestations of lesions of the suprasellar and parasellar regions: a neuro-ophthalmologic perspective. *Semin Ultrasound CT MR* **14**:206–214.

18. Garas G, Choudhury N, Farrell R. (2010) Invasive fatal rhino-orbito-cerebral mucormycosis in diabetic ketoacidosis. *JRSM Short Rep* **1**:57.

19. Almuhaideb A, Papathanasiou N, Bomanji J. (2011) 18F-FDG PET/CT imaging in oncology. *Ann Saudi Med* **31**:3–13.

20. Mostard RL, Van Kuijk SM, Verschakelen JA, *et al.* (2012) A predictive tool for an effective use of (18)F-FDG PET in assessing activity of sarcoidosis. *BMC Pulm Med* **12**:57.

21. Trouth JA, Dabi A, Solieman N, *et al.* (2012) Myasthenia gravis: a review. *Autoimmune Dis* **2012**:874680.

22. Browning J, Wallace M, Chana J, Booth J. (2011) Bedside testing for myasthenia gravis: the ice-test. *Emerg Med J* **28**:709–711.

23. Kim K, Kim MJ, Ahn S, *et al.* (2011) Frontal sinus lymphoma presenting as progressive multiple cranial nerve palsy. *Yonsei Med J* **52**:1044–1047.

24. Tsai RK, He MS, Cheu CL, Sheu MM. (2008) Transient third cranial nerve palsy caused by sphenoid sinus aspergillosis. *J Neuroophthalmol* **28**:239–240.

14

Cavernous Sinus Syndrome

Arielle Spitze MD, Lauren Jeang BA, Nagham Al-Zubidi MD,
Sushma Yalamanchili MD, and Andrew G. Lee MD

CASE

A 92-year-old Caucasian female presented with a one-day history of right-sided facial numbness, headache, and binocular, horizontal, and vertical (oblique) diplopia. Past medical history was notable for uterine cancer 30 years prior (treated surgically and in remission), stable, longstanding migraine headaches, and cardiac disease requiring pacemaker placement. External examination revealed right-sided numbness in the V_1 and V_2 distribution, but no facial asymmetry and good orbicularis oculi function bilaterally. Visual acuity was 20/30 in the right eye (OD) and 20/25 in the left eye (OS). Pupils measured 1.5 mm in the dark and 1 mm in the light in both eyes (OU) with no relative afferent pupillary defect. Visual fields were full to confrontation OU. Ocular motility examination revealed complete ophthalmoplegia OD, but normal motility OS (see Fig. 14.1). Corneal sensation was also decreased OD. Slit lamp examination was normal OU. Intraocular pressure measurements and dilated fundus examinations were normal OU. Magnetic resonance imaging (MRI) was unable to be performed due to the patient's pacemaker. Computed tomography (CT) and computed tomography angiography (CTA) showed bilateral cavernous sinus aneurysms and partially thrombosed and calcified distal internal carotid arterial aneurysms in the cavernous segments measuring 2.8 cm on the right and 2.5 cm on the left (see Fig. 14.2).

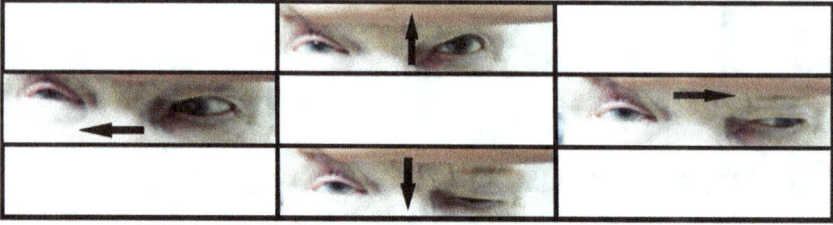

Fig. 14.1. Montage of photographs showing complete right-eye ophthalmoplegia. The right upper eyelid is being held open by an assistant. There was complete ptosis of the right eye in primary gaze.

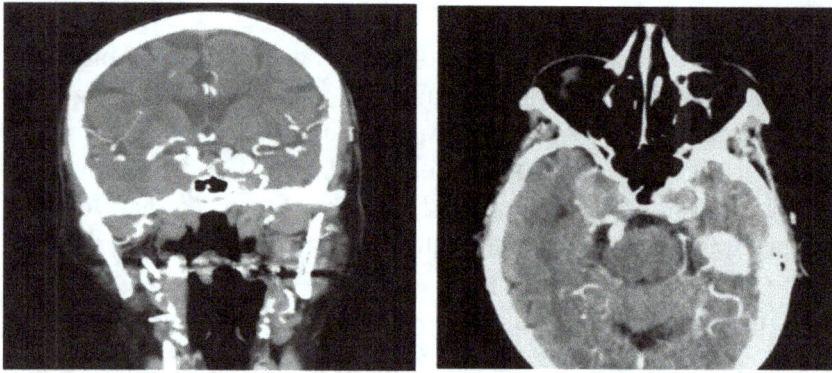

Fig. 14.2. Coronal and axial CTA revealing bilateral cavernous sinus aneurysms and partially thrombosed and calcified distal internal carotid arterial aneurysms in the cavernous segments measuring 2.8 cm on the right and 2.5 cm on the left. The cavernous sinus aneurysms were creating a mass-occupying lesion within the right-sided cavernous sinus, causing the patient to present with right cavernous sinus syndrome.

Question 1	Question 2
Which of the following additional signs is most likely to be present in a patient with an ipsilateral complete ophthalmoplegia due to a cavernous sinus lesion?	Which of the following tumors is least likely to be a cause of cavernous sinus syndrome?
A. Paresthesias in V_3 B. Numbness in cranial nerve V_{1-3} C. Horner syndrome D. Optic neuropathy	A. Pituitary adenoma B. Meningioma C. Pinealoma D. Craniopharyngioma
Question 3	**Question 4**
In a patient with a chronic, progressive, painless cavernous sinus syndrome, which of the following would be the best initial imaging study?	Which of the following infections is most likely to cause a cavernous sinus syndrome?
A. Contrast MRI of the head and orbit B. Contrast CT with CTA of the brain C. Digital subtraction angiography D. Contrast CT of the head and orbit	A. Otitis externa B. Encephalitis C. Endophthalmitis D. Sphenoid sinusitis
Question 5	**Question 6**
Which of the following cranial nerves is not involved in a typical cavernous sinus syndrome?	Which is the most vulnerable (and often first) nerve to become involved in a lesion of the substance of the cavernous sinus?
A. Cranial nerve II B. Cranial nerve III C. Cranial nerve IV D. Cranial nerve VI	A. Cranial nerve II B. Cranial nerve III C. Cranial nerve IV D. Cranial nerve VI

Question 7	Question 8
Which of the following MRI findings is most suggestive of infection-induced thrombosis of the cavernous sinus in an immunocompromised diabetic patient?	**Based on the most commonly identified pathogen in cavernous sinus thrombosis, which of the following would be the best initial intravenous treatment?**
A. Diffuse enhancement of the cavernous sinus and adjacent sphenoid sinus **B.** A rim-enhancing lesion within the sella turcica and T1 pre-contrast hyperintensity **C.** A homogeneously enhancing extra-axial mass with a dural tail **D.** A heterogeneously enhancing lesion in the sella with calcification and cysts	**A.** Vancomycin **B.** Cefepime **C.** Metronidazole **D.** Amphotericin B

EXPLANATIONS

The solution to Question 1 is C.

The cavernous sinus lies on either side of the sella turcica and is formed by the temporal and sphenoid bones of the skull. Cavernous sinus syndromes result from lesions (e.g., neoplasm, infection, inflammation, vascular) affecting structures in the cavernous sinus, which includes cranial nerves (CN) III, IV, V_1, V_2, VI, the intracavernous portion of the carotid artery, and postganglionic sympathetic fibers. Patients with cavernous sinus syndrome can present with partial or complete ophthalmoplegia (CN III, IV, VI), Horner syndrome (sympathetic fiber disruption), and sensory loss along the ophthalmic and maxillary nerves (CN V_1 and $V_{2,}$ respectively). Sensory loss along the mandible is not seen in cavernous sinus syndrome because the mandibular nerve (CN V_3) lies laterally to the cavernous sinus and is not contained within the cavernous sinus. Since the cavernous sinus is the only location where sympathetic fibers run closely with CN VI, an abduction deficit and esotropia with an ipsilateral Horner syndrome points towards cavernous sinus syndrome.[1] Horner syndrome, which is characterized by ipsilateral ptosis, miosis, and anhidrosis, can be often masked by levator muscle palsy from concurrent CN III palsy.[2] Orbicularis weakness, however, is caused by disruption to CN VII or myasthenia gravis. Since CN VII does not travel within the cavernous sinus, involvement of CN VII would not be expected to occur in cavernous sinus syndrome. Similarly, optic neuropathy would not be expected in cavernous sinus syndrome because the optic nerve travels through the optic canal and not the cavernous sinus. However, optic neuropathy may occur with extension of cavernous sinus lesions to the orbital apex or superior orbital fissure.

The solution to Question 2 is C.

Historically, in the pre-antibiotic era, infection was a common cause of cavernous sinus syndrome. However, with the prevalent use of antibiotics today, neoplasms, aneurysms, and carotid-cavernous fistulas are more common causes[3] and neoplasm is now the leading cause of cavernous sinus syndrome.[1,4,5] Neoplastic causes include metastatic disease from breast, lymphoma, lung, or prostate cancer[6]; primary tumors such as meningiomas, neurofibromas, and chondromas[5,7]; and local spread secondary from adjacent nasopharyngeal or pituitary tumors including pituitary adenomas and pituitary apoplexy.[5,7] Pituitary tumors can be associated with endocrine symptoms such as galactorrhea, acromegaly, and hypopituitarism, which can help confirm the clinical diagnosis.[1] Although older studies found nasopharyngeal cancer to be a common lesion,[8,9] a recent study of 150 operated cases suggested that meningiomas are the most common type of tumor affecting the cavernous sinus.[10] Another study of 126 patients found pituitary adenomas and meningiomas to be most common.[5] Rarer causes of cavernous sinus syndrome can include Tolosa–Hunt syndrome (idiopathic granulomatous disease),[11] herpes zoster,[12] sarcoidosis,[13] and trauma.[4] In contrast, a pinealoma is a tumor of the pineal gland, which is located more posteriorly near the dorsal midbrain. Thus, a pinealoma would be unlikely to directly affect the cavernous sinus. Rather, symptoms of a pinealoma are more likely to present as a dorsal midbrain syndrome (i.e., upgaze palsy, convergence-retraction nystagmus, light-near dissociation, and eyelid retraction).

The solution to Question 3 is A.

MRI is the best imaging modality for mass lesions while CTA is better for vascular pathologies such as thrombosis, aneurysms, and fistulas.[1] A slow-growing, painless, progressive lesion would be most suggestive of a neoplasm rather than vascular lesion. Thus, an MRI of the head and orbit with and without gadolinium would need to be performed to reveal any neoplastic or other contrast-enhancing lesions such as an intracavernous menigioma. The orbit should be included to evaluate for any involvement or extension from the cavernous sinus into the orbital apex. Digital subtraction angiography (DSA) is useful to further define morphologies and flow patterns seen on CTA.[1] DSA, however, has been largely replaced by CTA and is not as commonly performed as a first line test to evaluate for the etiology of a cavernous sinus syndrome. If a vascular lesion is suspected and not well visualized on MRI or CTA, then DSA could be performed.

The solution to Question 4 is D.

The cavernous sinus receives blood from the superior and inferior ophthalmic veins, cerebral veins, and the sphenoparietal sinus. It then drains through the superior and inferior petrosal sinuses into the jugular vein. It is also connected to the pterygoid plexus via the inferior ophthalmic vein, deep facial vein, and emissary vein. Due to its extensive connections to the facial vein via the ophthalmic veins, the cavernous sinus is vulnerable to infections from the facial danger triangle, or the area which contains the corners of the mouth and the nose. These infections, in turn, can spread to the brain. Mortality from cavernous sinus thrombosis used to be nearly 100% but now is lower (20–30% or less) due to current advances in antibiotic treatment.[14]

Sphenoid and ethmoid sinusitis are the most common causes of cavernous sinus thrombophlebitis and infectious cavernous sinus thrombosis, which both can present with a cavernous sinus syndrome.[14] Other causes of infectious spread that can lead to cavernous sinus thrombosis include otitis media, parotitis, mastoiditis, tonsillitis, dental caries, and septic emboli arising from the facial veins secondary to infections of the face.[3,14,15] Despite receiving drainage from the ophthalmic veins, cavernous sinus thrombosis is rarely caused by ocular infections[14] (i.e., endophthalmitis). Neither otitis externa nor encephalitis would be expected to cause infectious cavernous sinus thrombosis.

The solution to Question 5 is A.

Involvement of CN II (the optic nerve) would not be expected in cavernous sinus syndrome, as the optic nerve travels through the optic canal, and not within the cavernous sinus. Rather, involvement of CN II would be expected to occur in orbital apex syndrome, which can affect any or all of the structures within the orbital apex (CN II, III, IV, V_1, VI). All of the structures within the orbital apex can also be affected in cavernous sinus syndrome, with the optic nerve as the only exception. However, the optic nerve could be secondarily affected in cavernous sinus syndrome due to increased venous pressure within the cavernous sinus and superior ophthalmic vein (disc edema or dilated retinal veins), although this can occur asymptomatically and may not necessarily cause vision loss. In addition, involvement of both the orbital apex and cavernous sinus can occur; however, vision loss would still be more consistent with orbital apex syndrome rather than cavernous sinus syndrome and imaging may be required to determine the exact lesion location.

The solution to Question 6 is D.

CN VI is often the first nerve to be affected in cavernous sinus syndrome because it is located in the medial aspect of the substance rather than the wall of the cavernous sinus. This position makes it more vulnerable to infection or compression from the surrounding vasculature. CN III, IV, V_1, and V_2 are located within the dural layers of the lateral wall of the cavernous sinus, which offers additional protection from injury; thus, they are normally affected later in the disease process.[3] CN II does not travel within the cavernous sinus, so it would not be expected to be involved in a typical cavernous sinus syndrome. However, CN II can be affected in select cases, such as with extension of cavernous sinus lesions into the orbital apex, or sellar lesions that extend laterally into the cavernous sinus and also superiorly to affect the optic chiasm (e.g., pituitary apoplexy).

The solution to Question 7 is A.

Diagnosing the etiology of cavernous sinus thrombosis secondary to bacterial or fungal infection depends largely on history, but certain findings on MRI may help. In general, cavernous sinus thrombosis will appear on imaging with cavernous sinus enlargement, dilated tributary veins including the ipsilateral superior ophthalmic vein, and exophthalmos.[16] Thrombosis caused by bacterial pathogens typically appears on MRI as diffuse enhancement because of surrounding tissue cellulitis and associated edema, which causes a breakdown in the blood-brain barrier, allowing contrast material to extravasate.[16] Actinomycosis, a bacterial infection commonly associated with immunocompromised and diabetic patients, often appears as a ring-enhancing abscess with irregular margins.[16] Mucormycosis and aspergillosis, which are also seen in immunocompromised and dia-betic patients, are infections resulting from fungi that usually enter via the nasal cavity and cause necrosis of vascular structures.[16] Typically adjacent sinusitis is a likely indicator of the origin of fungal infection. The lesions can also appear on MRI as non-enhancing lesions with vascular necrosis. Tolosa–Hunt syndrome, an idiopathic non-caseating granulomatous inflammation causing painful ophthalmoplegia, will appear on MRI as a contrast-enhancing homogeneous area of cavernous sinus enhancement.[16] Patients with Tolosa–Hunt syndrome would also report improvement with corticosteroids, unlike in an infectious process, where corticosteroids would be detrimental. Thus, the clinician should be cautious about making the diagnosis of idiopathic or inflammatory disease in immunosuppressed or diabetic patients in whom fungal disease is a consideration. A meningioma often appears on MRI as an isointense extra-axial mass with homogeneous enhancement and a dural tail. Pituitary apoplexy on MRI typically shows an intrasellar mass with a rim of hyperintensity on precontrast T1 suggestive of blood and an enhancing rim of tissue surrounding a necrotic hypointense or hemorrhagic variable-intensity core. A craniopharyngioma typically appears as a heterogeneous, solid, and cystic suprasellar lesion with variable enhancement on MRI.

The solution to Question 8 is A.

The most common pathogen causing infectious cavernous sinus thrombosis is methicillin-susceptible *Staphylococcus aureus* (MSSA), but community-acquired methicillin-resistant *S. aureus* (MRSA) is becoming increasingly common.[14,17] For adults with MRSA thrombosis, the Infectious Diseases Society of America guidelines are for intravenous (IV) vancomycin for four to six weeks with the possible addition of rifampin to increase concentrations in the cerebrospinal fluid.[18] Surgical drainage is recommended only if it can be done safely, but this is rare.[9,18] IV nafcillin is also used for MSSA infection, cefepime is often used for pseudomonas infection, and metronidazole for anaerobic coverage. Amphotericin B is reserved for fungal infections. Use of heparin anti-coagulation therapy and steroids in conjunction with antibiotic therapy is still debated.[14,18–20]

SUMMARY

Cavernous sinus syndrome is characterized by variable findings of partial or complete ophthalmoplegia, ptosis, Horner syndrome, and sensory loss along the trigeminal branches (ophthalmic and maxillary divisions). These signs correspond to a disruption in any combination of CN III, IV, V_1, V_2, VI, or the oculosympathetic nerves. A sixth nerve palsy with a concomitant Horner syndrome is a classic combination of findings suggesting cavernous sinus syndrome. Other systemic signs may be present in acute cavernous sinus lesions, including headache, fever, periorbital swelling, proptosis, and chemosis. The infectious or inflammatory cavernous sinus syndrome can be mistaken for orbital cellulitis, but bilateral eye involvement, pupil involvement without visual loss, and periocular sensory loss are key differentiators. Neoplasm is a common cause of chronic or progressive cavernous sinus syndrome. Other less common causes include intracavernous carotid artery aneurysms, carotid-cavernous fistulas, infections, trauma, Tolosa–Hunt syndrome, herpes zoster, and sarcoidosis. Imaging with MRI and CT are most helpful in the diagnosis and the combination of studies may be necessary in evaluating cavernous sinus lesions. Septic thrombosis of the cavernous sinus, also known as cavernous sinus thrombophlebitis, was once a frequent deadly complication of facial infections, but it has become less common today due to antibiotics. *Staphylococcus aureus* is a common cause of infectious cavernous sinus thrombophlebitis and thus the recommended initial empiric treatment is IV vancomycin for MRSA or IV nafcillin for MSSA.

REFERENCES

1. Bone I, Hadley DM. (2005) Syndromes of the orbital fissure, cavernous sinus, cerebellopontine angle, and skull base. *J Neurol Neurosurg Psychiatry* **76 Suppl 3**:iii29–iii38.
2. Duong DK, Leo MM, Mitchell EL. (2008) Neuro-ophthalmology. *Emerg Med Clin North Am* **26**:137–180.

3. Van Overbeeke JJ, Jansen JJ, Tulleken CA. (1988) The cavernous sinus syndrome. An anatomical and clinical study. *Clin Neurol Neurosurg* **90**:311–319.

4. Keane JR. (1996) Cavernous sinus syndrome: analysis of 151 cases. *Arch Neurol* **53**:967–971.

5. Fernández S, Godino O, Martinez-Yelamos S, *et al.* (2007) Cavernous sinus syndrome: a series of 126 patients. *Medicine (Baltimore)* **86**:278–281.

6. Spell DW, Gervais DS Jr, Ellis JK, Vial RH. (1998) Cavernous sinus syndrome due to metastatic renal cell carcinoma. *South Med J* **91**:576–579.

7. Lazino G, Hirsch WL, Pomonis S, *et al.* (1992) Cavernous sinus tumors: neuro-radiologic and neurosurgical considerations on 150 operated cases. *J Neurosurg Sci* **36**:183–196.

8. Thomas JE, Yoss RE. (1970) The parasellar syndrome: problems in determining etiology. *Mayo Clin Proc* **45**:617–623.

9. Newman S. (2007) A prospective study of cavernous sinus surgery for meningi-omas and resultant common ophthalmic complications (an American Ophthalmological Society thesis). *Trans Am Ophthalmol Soc* **105**:392–447.

10. Hirsch WL, Sekhar LN, Lanzino G, *et al.* (1993) Meningiomas involving the cavernous sinus: value of imaging for predicting surgical complications. *AJR Am J Roentgenol* **160**:1083–1088.

11. Leijzer CTJM, Prevo RL, Hageman G. (1999) Meningioma presenting as Tolosa–Hunt syndrome. *Clin Neurol Neurosurg* **101**:19–22.

12. Motohiro N, Toshio K, Yuichi O, *et al.* (2002) A case of cavernous sinus syn-drome following herpes zoster ophthalmicus. *Folia Ophthalmologica Japonica* **53**:898–903.

13. Chang C-S, Chen W-L, Li CT, Wang PY. (2009) Cavernous sinus syndrome due to sarcoidosis: a case report. *Acta Neurol Taiwan* **18**:37–41.

14. Ebright JR, Pace MT, Niazi AF. (2001) Septic thrombosis of the cavernous sinuses. *Arch Intern Med* **161**:2671–2676.

15. Chow AW. (1992) Life-threatening infections of the head and neck. *Clin Infect Dis* **14**:991–1002.

16. Lee JH, Lee HK, Park JK, *et al.* (2003) Cavernous sinus syndrome: clinical fea-tures and differential diagnosis with MR imaging. *AJR Am J Roentgenol* **181**:583–590.

17. Southwick FS, Richardson EP Jr, Swartz MN. (1986) Septic thrombosis of the dural venous sinuses. *Medicine (Baltimore)* **65**:82–106.

18. Liu C, Bayer A, Cosgrove SE, *et al.* (2011) Clinical practice guidelines by the Infectious Diseases Society of America for the treatment of methicillin-resistant Staphylococcus aureus infections in adults and children. *Clin Infect Dis* **52**:e18–e55.

19. Levine SR, Twyman RE, Gilman S. (1988) The role of anticoagulation in cavern-ous sinus thrombosis. *Neurology* **38**:517–522.

20. Tsai FY, Kostanian V, Rivera M, *et al.* (2007) Cerebral venous congestion as indication for thrombolytic treatment. *Cardiovasc Intervent Radiol* **30**:675–687.

15

Arteriovenous Anomalies — Carotid-Cavernous Fistula

Arielle Spitze MD, Megha Agrawal MD, Nagham Al-Zubidi MD, Sushma Yalamanchili MD, and Andrew G. Lee MD

CASE

A 53-year-old Caucasian male presented with six weeks of acute-onset painless binocular vertical diplopia. He then developed proptosis, lid edema, redness, and a pulsatile sensation in the right eye (OD). His past medical history was significant only for medication-controlled hyperlipidemia, and he denied a history of hypertension, diabetes, or trauma. The remainder of his medical history was unremarkable. On examination, he had moderate lower lid edema OD but no lid retraction or lid lag. Hertel measurements showed 5 mm of proptosis OD. His best-corrected visual acuity was 20/20 in both eyes (OU). The pupillary exam was normal and there was no relative afferent pupillary defect (RAPD). Extraocular movements showed slight adduction and elevation deficits OD. There was a moderate right exotropia and right hypertropia that was worse on right head tilt. The intraocular pressure was 20 mmHg OD and 15 mmHg in the left eye (OS). Markedly pulsatile and wide mires were noted OD as compared to normal applanation mires OS. Slit lamp examination showed arterialized, tortuous, and dilated conjunctival vessels extending to the limbus OD (see Fig. 15.1), but biomicroscopy was normal OS. Dilated funduscopic exam showed mildly dilated veins OD but was otherwise normal OU. Automated visual fields (Humphrey 24-2) were normal OU. Magnetic resonance imaging (MRI) of the brain and orbits with and without gadolinium with

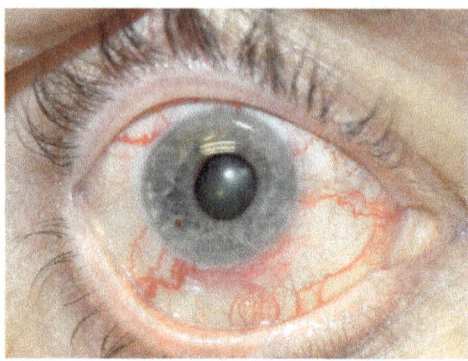

Fig. 15.1. External photograph shows the arterialized, tortuous, dilated conjunctival vessels extending to the limbus. This is the differentiating sign of a CCF on slit lamp exam. Note the intervening clear zones of conjunctiva.

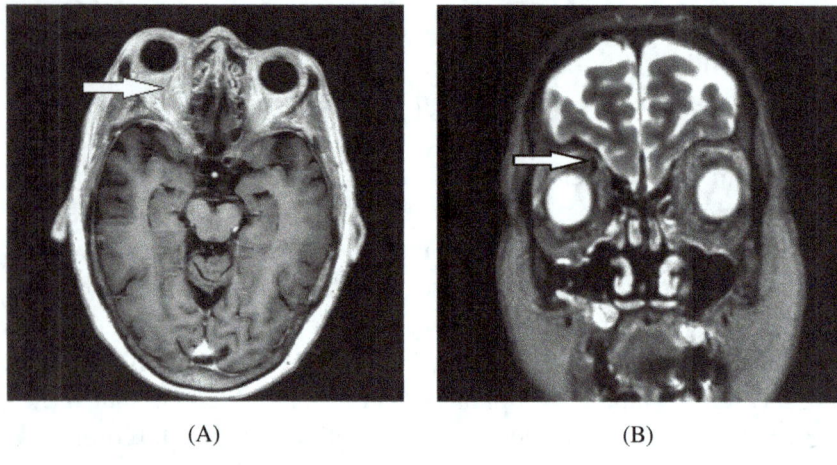

(A)   (B)

Fig. 15.2. Axial T1 post-contrast with fat saturation (A) and coronal post-contrast T2 image with fat saturation (B) demonstrating an enlarged right SOV (arrow). This is a distinctive sign of a CCF on MRI that is due to retrograde venous flow. The SOV also demonstrates an arterialized flow void (dark signal on T2).

fat suppression demonstrated an enlarged right superior ophthalmic vein (SOV) and inferior ophthalmic vein with arterial flow voids present in these normally slow-flow veins (see Fig. 15.2). A cerebral catheter angiogram showed an indirect dural arteriovenous (AV) fistula of the right cavernous sinus supplied by branches of the internal and external carotid arteries (see Fig. 15.3).

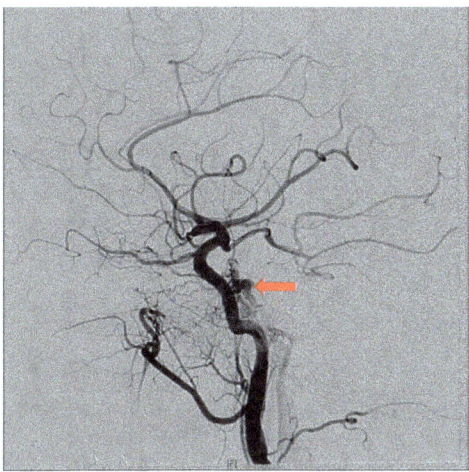

Fig. 15.3. Cerebral catheter angiogram demonstrates an indirect dural carotid-cavernous AV fistula supplied by branches of the right internal and external carotid arteries (Barrow classification type D). In this image, the drainage pattern is mostly posterior (draining from the cavernous sinus down the inferior petrosal sinus (arrow)).

Question 1	Question 2
Which of the following describes the Barrow classification of a fistula arising directly from the internal carotid artery and communicating with the cavernous sinus?	Which of the following is a distinctive sign of a patient presenting with a suspected high-flow carotid-cavernous fistula (CCF)?
A. Type A **B.** Type B **C.** Type C **D.** Type D	**A.** Lid retraction **B.** Ophthalmoplegia **C.** Proptosis **D.** Audible bruit

Question 3	Question 4
Which of the following is a differentiating sign of CCF on slit lamp examination?	**Which of the following imaging studies is the gold standard for the diagnosis of a CCF?**
A. Superior limbic keratoconjunctivitis **B.** Arterialization of conjunctival vessels **C.** Conjunctival chemosis **D.** Prominent iris vessels	**A.** Computed tomography (CT) of the brain **B.** MRI of the brain with MR angiography (MRA) **C.** Cerebral catheter angiogram **D.** CT angiography (CTA) of the brain
Question 5	**Question 6**
Which of the following is the distinctive radiographic sign of a CCF on orbital color Doppler ultrasound?	**Which of the following is the most urgent indication for endovascular treatment of a CCF?**
A. Asymmetric superior ophthalmic vein **B.** Anterograde flow in the orbital veins **C.** Diminished flow in the internal or external carotid artery **D.** Enlarged internal or external carotid artery	**A.** Diplopia and ophthalmoplegia **B.** Elevated intraocular pressure **C.** Retinal venous dilation **D.** Cortical venous drainage
Question 7	**Question 8**
Which of the following is the best treatment for a chronic symptomatic CCF?	**Which of the following causes of vision loss describes a mechanism occurring directly from a CCF?**
A. Surgical carotid artery sacrifice **B.** External beam radiation **C.** Carotid massage **D.** Endovascular embolization	**A.** Low intraocular pressure **B.** Compressive optic neuropathy **C.** Central retinal vein occlusion **D.** Chiasmal compression

EXPLANATIONS

The solution to Question 1 is A.

Carotid-cavernous fistulas (CCFs) arise from anomalous connections between branches of the carotid arterial system and the cavernous sinus.[1,2]

CCFs can be angiographically classified according to the Barrow classification.[3] A Barrow type A CCF is a direct, high-flow communication between the intracavernous internal carotid artery (ICA) and the cavernous sinus. Trauma, including motor vehicle accidents, falls, and penetrating head and orbit injuries, account for 70–90% of this type of CCF. Type A CCFs can also be caused iatrogenically in procedures such as carotid angioplasties or transsphenoidal procedures, or from rupture of an underlying intracavernous aneurysm. When secondary to trauma, type A fistulas often develop immediately or within a few days to weeks after the initial injury. In contrast, Barrow type B fistulas are branches of the ICA communicating with the cavernous sinus. Type C CCFs are due to branches of the external carotid artery (ECA) communicating with the cavernous sinus. Type D fistulas occur when branches of both the ICA and ECA communicate with the cavernous sinus. Barrow types B–D are considered indirect or dural, low-flow carotid-cavernous fistulas. Type B is the least common type of CCF, while type D is the most common type. In contrast to a typical high-flow, type A CCF, most indirect fistulas occur insidiously when small dural arteries spontaneously rupture, typically in middle-aged females with hypertension.[1–3]

The solution to Question 2 is D.

Direct, type A fistulas tend to be high-flow CCFs due to direct tears in the ICA, while indirect fistulas are typically low-flow CCFs.[1–4] Most high-flow CCFs and even some lower-flow CCFs may produce an audible subjective bruit heard by the patient or by the physician with a stethoscope (using the bell placed over the orbit or head).[2,4] This bruit is very specific to CCFs and other disorders are much less likely if an audible bruit is present. Lid retraction is a sign of thyroid eye disease. Other signs that can be found with a CCF such as edema, ophthalmoplegia, proptosis, or chemosis, and other less specific symptoms of high- and low-flow CCFs (binocular diplopia, conjunctival injection, edematous or ptotic eyelids, and ipsilateral facial or retrobulbar pain), can overlap with those found in other conditions such as thyroid eye disease, orbital infectious processes, orbital inflammatory disorders, or orbital neoplasms.[2]

The solution to Question 3 is B.

Retrograde flow of blood from the high-pressure arterial system to the lower-pressure venous system in the orbit (via the SOV) may result in dilated and tortuous or corkscrew-shaped episcleral and conjunctival blood vessels (i.e., arterialized flow) approaching the limbus. Superior limbic keratoconjunctivitis would be more suggestive of thyroid eye disease, and not a CCF. While conjunctival chemosis and prominent iris vessels can occur in CCFs, they are non-specific findings and are not distinctive of a CCF. Arterialized episcleral and conjunctival vessels are a distinctive and differentiating (although not universal) finding on slit lamp examination of patients with CCFs and are a typical finding in the anterior draining CCF (i.e., the red-eyed shunt). In contrast, posterior flow of the arterialized blood from the cavernous sinus draining into the inferior petrosal sinus may not produce the typical anterior features of proptosis, injection, chemosis, and arterialized episcleral and conjunctival vessels. Instead, the patient with this so-called posterior draining CCF (i.e., the white-eyed shunt) may be asymptomatic from an ophthalmological standpoint or only present with subtle findings. For example, these patients may only have chronic ipsilateral pain and ophthalmoplegia (typically sixth nerve palsy); thus, a high index of suspicion is necessary to make the diagnosis, as neuroimaging may be negative and the typical and distinctive radiographic sign for the anterior draining CCF (i.e., enlarged SOV) may be absent in the posterior draining CCF. Interestingly, progression from a white-eyed shunt to a red-eyed shunt may also occur and may require more urgent treatment as the blood flow pattern changes from posterior to anterior drainage.[2,5]

In an anterior draining CCF, the increased venous pressure may produce lid or periorbital edema, and in severe cases, corneal ulceration secondary to exposure or neurotrophic keratopathy may occur. Increased intraocular pressure with widely pulsating mires during applanation tonometry may also be a helpful sign if present.[1,2,4,5]

Auscultation of the globe or temple may reveal a bruit, but as noted above, this sign is typically absent in low-flow fistulas and its absence does not exclude the diagnosis of a CCF.[2,4] Diplopia may result either from involvement of cranial nerve (CN) III, IV, or VI as they pass through the cavernous sinus, or from extraocular muscle ischemia or edema.[1,2] Likewise, neurogenic or mechanical ptosis may occur in CCFs. Involvement of CN III or the sympathetic pathway within the cavernous sinus can also lead to anisocoria with ipsilateral mydriasis (CN III) or miosis (Horner syndrome), respectively.[2] Involvement of CN V_1 or V_2 may result in facial numbness or pain.[1]

The solution to Question 4 is C.

Although cranial contrast CT scan, CTA, MRI, MRA, orbital ultrasonography, and transorbital/transcranial color Doppler imaging may all reveal findings in support of a suspected CCF, cerebral catheter angiogram remains the gold standard diagnostic test for a CCF. Selective angiography of both the ICA and ECA bilaterally is also highly recommended for full classification of a CCF, for identifying feeding vessels and venous drainage (including cortical drainage), and for guiding possible endovascular treatment.[1,2] Initial imaging with CT or MRI of the head and orbit with and without contrast (with or without CTA or MRA) is the initial recommended imaging study for a CCF and might show the diagnostic radiographic feature of the dilated superior ophthalmic vein. In addition, structural neuroimaging can show evidence for intracranial ischemia or hemorrhage and can exclude other conditions that might mimic a CCF clinically.

The solution to Question 5 is B.

In the CCF, anterograde, arterialized flow is transmitted from the carotid arterial circulation through the cavernous sinus and anteriorly to the inferior and superior ophthalmic veins. This arterialization of orbital venous outflow produces the distinctive clinical and radiographic sign of the CCF (i.e., an enlarged SOV). Arterialized flow can sometimes also be seen in the SOV or other orbital veins on orbital color Doppler ultrasound and may be visible as a flow void on conventional MRI (see Fig. 15.2). The increased flow in the cavernous sinus may also be seen as intracavernous arterial flow voids or fullness in the cavernous sinus.[1]

The solution to Question 6 is D.

Worsening vision, diplopia, ophthalmoplegia, intolerable bruit, or severe proptosis resulting in exposure keratopathy may all be indications for interventional treatment of a CCF. Cortical venous drainage, however, (best visualized on catheter arteriography) is a particularly dangerous finding. These patients are at higher risk for cerebral venous infarction or hemorrhage due to elevated intracranial venous pressure. Patients with cortical venous drainage should therefore undergo neuroradiological intervention and treatment. In contrast, other patients with low-flow dural CCFs, mild ocular symptoms, and no high-risk features on angiography for hemorrhage or venous infarction may be observed for spontaneous closure, which has been reported in approximately 20–50% of patients.[2] Patients with CCFs should, however, be monitored with regular ocular examinations, including visual acuity, visual fields, pupil, motility, exophthalmometry, and intraocular pressure (IOP) measurements, as well as dilated fundus examinations. Stable, mild diplopia may be managed initially with prisms or patching. Elevated IOP often responds to topical or oral aqueous suppressants. Since the mechanism of increased IOP is due to increased episcleral venous pressure, topical medications that increase outflow, such as prostaglandin analogs and cholinergic agonists, are less effective. If the elevated IOP is refractory to medical therapy, it typically resolves with CCF endovascular or spontaneous closure.[2]

The solution to Question 7 is D.

In contrast to high-flow, direct (type A) CCFs which generally require interventional therapy, observation alone may result in spontaneous closure of a low-flow dural CCF in 20–50% of patients.[2] In addition, some dural CCFs also close spontaneously with intermittent manual external self-occlusion of the ipsilateral carotid artery. In this technique, the internal carotid artery is occluded temporarily using the contralateral hand to avoid prolonged ischemia (because if ischemic hemiparesis were to develop from the ipsilateral ICA, the occluding hand would fall away from the neck). Other cases of CCFs have closed spontaneously after catheter arteriography alone.[1]

Endovascular embolization is the treatment of choice for most CCFs. Transarterial or transvenous embolization (including the direct superior ophthalmic vein approach) with detachable balloon or other occlusive materials (e.g., glue, coil, Onyx) may result in successful long-term fistula obliteration in 90–100% of cases.[1,2,4,6–9] Although there are some risks of endovascular treatment, in general this procedure has low morbidity and mortality.[1,2,8,9]

The solution to Question 8 is C.

Untreated direct, high-flow CCFs have a high morbidity and potential mortality and can result in epistaxis, intracerebral hemorrhage, and death. Visual loss can also occur in both untreated direct and indirect CCFs from a variety of mechanisms, including (but not limited to) central retinal vein occlusion, ischemic optic neuropathy, glaucoma, and chorioretinal dysfunction.[2] Every mechanism of visual loss from a CCF is directly or indirectly related to increased venous pressure, but some occur through a direct action and some indirectly. Central retinal vein occlusion would occur as a direct result of increased venous pressure in the orbital veins and is therefore a direct mechanism of vision loss occurring from a CCF. In contrast, a CCF would not cause a compressive optic neuropathy because the optic nerve does not pass within the cavernous sinus; however, an ischemic optic neuropathy could indirectly occur from increased venous pressure leading to decreased oxygen supplying the optic nerve. Similarly, increased intraocular pressure (glaucoma with secondary glaucomatous optic neuropathy) could be related to a CCF, but would be an indirect mechanism of vision loss since the increased venous pressure leads to decreased aqueous reabsorption, which therefore leads to increased intraocular pressure. In contrast, a CCF would not cause low intraocular pressure-related vision loss (i.e., hypotony maculopathy). Chiasmal compression is most commonly caused by tumors of the pituitary gland and would not normally occur with a CCF.

SUMMARY

Indirect, low-flow CCFs may develop spontaneously, typically in hypertensive women over 50 years old. Direct (type A), high-flow fistulas often result from trauma, occult intracavernous aneurysm rupture, or iatrogenically after invasive surgical procedures. Patients with anterior draining CCFs (red-eyed shunts) typically present with proptosis, elevated IOP, ophthalmoplegia, diplopia, and the distinctive clinical sign of arterialization of the conjunctival and episcleral blood vessels. The gold standard diagnostic test is catheter angiogram, but a CT or MRI of the head and orbit may show the distinctive radiographic sign of an enlarged superior (or less commonly inferior) ophthalmic vein. Orbital ultrasound may demonstrate reversal of blood flow and arterialization of the SOV. Without treatment, direct CCFs may lead to morbidity or mortality, including vision loss in up to 80–90% of patients. Thus, these high-flow CCFs typically require treatment. Endovascular embolization results in long-term fistula obliteration in most patients (90–100%). In contrast, indirect CCF patients with mild ocular symptoms may be observed and managed symptomatically or with intermittent manual carotid occlusion. For markedly symptomatic patients (e.g., those with intolerable bruit, ophthalmoplegia, severe intractable glaucoma, or visual loss), or those with cortical venous drainage demonstrated on catheter angiography, the practitioner should strongly consider treatment with endovascular embolization.

REFERENCES

1. Shownkeen H, Boya D, Origitano T, *et al.* (2001) Carotid-cavernous fistulas: pathogenesis and routes of approach to endovascular treatment. *Skull Base* **11**:207–218.
2. Miller NR. (2007) Diagnosis and management of dural carotid-cavernous sinus fistulas. *Neurosurg Focus* **23**:E13.
3. Barrow DL, Spector RH, Braun IF, *et al.* (1985) Classification and treatment of spontaneous carotid cavernous sinus fistulas. *J Neurosurg* **62**:248–256.
4. Lewis AI, Tomsick TA, Tew JM Jr. (1995) Management of 100 consecutive direct carotid-cavernous fistulas: results of treatment with detachable balloons. *Neurosurgery* **36**:239–245.
5. Stiebel-Kalish H, Setton A, Nimii Y, *et al.* (2002) Cavernous sinus dural arterio-venous malformations: patterns of venous drainage are related to clinical signs and symptoms. *Ophthalmology* **109**:1685–1691.
6. Wang W, Li YD, Li MH, *et al.* (2011) Endovascular treatment of post-traumatic direct carotid-cavernous fistulas: a single-center experience. *J Clin Neurosci* **18**:24–28.
7. Keltner JL, Satterfield D, Dublin AB, Lee BC. (1987) Dural and carotid cavernous fistulas: diagnosis, management and complications. *Ophthalmology* **94**:1585–1600.
8. Meyers PM, Halbach VV, Dowd CF, *et al.* (2002) Dural carotid cavernous fistula: definitive endovascular management and long-term follow-up. *Am J Ophthalmol* **134**:85–92.
9. Gupta AK, Purkayastha S, Krishnamoorthy T, *et al.* (2006) Endovascular treatment of direct carotid cavernous fistulae: a pictorial review. *Neuroradiology* **48**: 831–839.

16

Chiasmal Disorders

Nagham Al-Zubidi MD, Whitlow Bryan Thomas BS,
Arielle Spitze MD, Sushma Yalamanchili MD, and
Andrew G. Lee MD

CASE

An 81-year-old man presented with four-month history of painless progressive bilateral loss of vision. He denied any history of headaches or other neurologic symptoms. The remainder of his past medical, surgical, social, family, and ocular history was negative. He was on no medication. His visual acuity was 20/20 in both eyes (OU). Ishihara color plate scoring was 0 out of 14 in the right eye (OD) and 2 out of 14 in the left eye (OS). Pupils were 3 mm in the dark and 2 mm in the light OU, and there was no relative afferent pupillary defect (RAPD) or light-near dissociation. Extraocular motility and intraocular pressure measurements were normal. Slit lamp biomicroscopy showed a posterior chamber intraocular lens OD and a mild nuclear sclerotic cataract OS. Automated (Humphrey 24-2) visual field testing is shown in (Fig. 16.1). The cup-to-disc ratio was 0.25 OU but there was significant temporal pallor OU. There was no disc edema. The rest of the funduscopic examination was normal. Magnetic resonance imaging (MRI) of the brain with and without contrast showed a large 4.6 cm × 2.9 cm × 3 cm mass with heterogeneous T2 signal, and enhancement in the sella, and suprasellar extension with compression of the optic chiasm from below (Fig. 16.2).

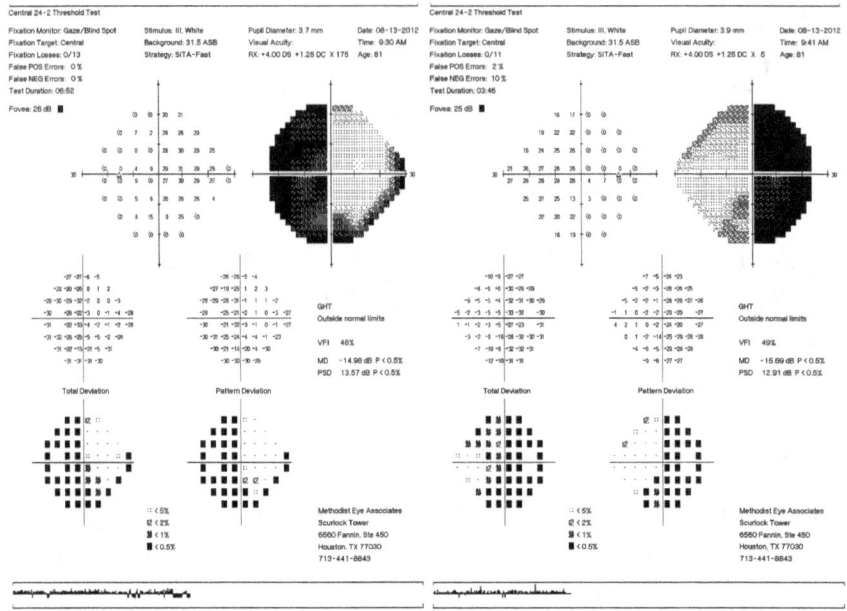

Fig. 16.1. Humphrey visual field 24-2 showing bitemporal hemianopsia.

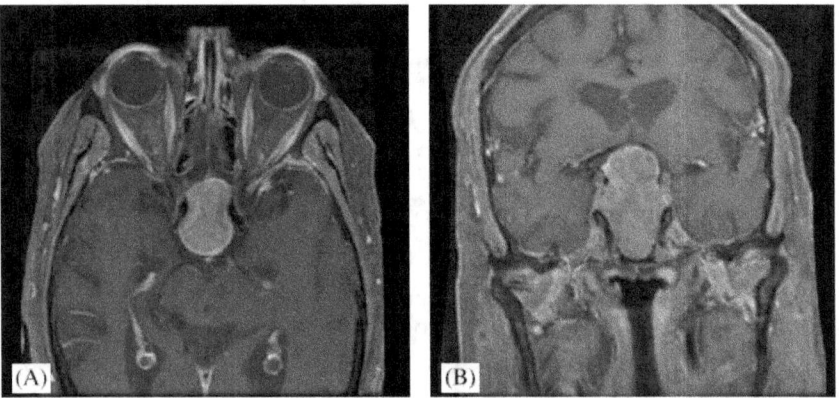

Fig. 16.2. MRI of the brain with contrast showing pituitary adenoma 4.6 × 2.9 × 3 cm sella /suprasellar compressing the optic chiasm. (A) Axial post-contrast. (B) Coronal post-contrast.

Question 1	Question 2
Which of the following is the most likely presenting finding of a typical pituitary adenoma?	**Which of the following is the most likely cause of a suprasellar lesion with the imaging characteristic shown in Fig. 16.2?**
A. Acute, painless, downbeat nystagmus **B.** Progressive bitemporal vision loss **C.** Acute, painful, isolated Horner syndrome **D.** Alternating, variable, and fatigable ptosis	**A.** Carotid artery aneurysm **B.** Sellar meningioma **C.** Pituitary adenoma **D.** Craniopharyngioma
Question 3	**Question 4**
Which of the following visual field defects is most likely with a body of the chiasm lesion?	**Which of the following visual field defects is most likely to be associated with a prefixed chiasmal anatomy?**
A. Bitemporal hemianopsia **B.** Junctional scotoma **C.** Cecocentral scotoma **D.** Homonymous hemianopsia	**A.** Bitemporal hemianopsia **B.** Junctional scotoma **C.** Bilateral cecocentral scotomas **D.** Homonymous hemianopsia
Question 5	**Question 6**
Which of the following diagnosis is the most likely cause of the visual field defect shown in Fig. 16.3?	**Which of the following is the best neuroradiologic study for the evaluation of a chronic chiasmal disorder?**
A. Myopic posterior staphyloma **B.** Pituitary adenoma **C.** Optic nerve head drusen **D.** Demyelinating optic neuritis	**A.** Computed tomography angiogram (CTA) of the head **B.** Cranial CT with and without contrast **C.** MRI of the orbit without contrast **D.** MRI of the brain with gadolinium

Question 7	Question 8
Which of the following suprasellar lesions requires urgent evaluation, management, and possible hospital admission?	Which of the following is the best treatment for a non-secreting pituitary adenoma with symptomatic compression of the optic chiasm?
A. Craniopharyngioma **B.** Meningioma **C.** Pituitary apoplexy **D.** Optic chiasmal glioma	**A.** Transsphenoidal surgery **B.** Bromocriptine therapy **C.** Bifrontal craniotomy **D.** Primary radiosurgery
Question 9	Question 10
Which of the following medical treatments is most likely to be beneficial in a symptomatic prolactin-secreting pituitary macroadenoma?	Which of the following is the most likely postsurgical prognosis for visual recovery for a patient with a pituitary adenoma and the OCT shown?
A. Dopamine antagonist **B.** Cholinergic agonist **C.** Dopamine agonist **D.** Serotonin agonist	**A.** No improvement **B.** Poor improvement **C.** Fair improvement **D.** Good improvement

EXPLANATIONS

The solution to Question 1 is B.

The majority of chronic optic chiasmal lesions in adults are caused by slowly growing neoplasms such as pituitary adenoma, craniopharyngioma, or meningioma. Dysgerminoma and optic chiasmal glioma can occur in younger patients, however. In addition, internal carotid suprasellar aneurysm can act as a mass lesion on the chiasm and may mimic a pituitary adenoma. The most common symptom of chiasmal compressive lesions is gradual, painless, progressive bilateral vision loss (typically bitemporal hemianopsia). The anatomy of the chiasm can affect whether the optic nerve (postfixed chiasm), body of the chiasm (typical anatomic configuration), or optic tract (prefixed chiasm) is affected by the suprasellar mass (see below). Acute painful bitemporal hemianopsia from chiasmal compressive lesions is highly suggestive of pituitary apoplexy caused by infarction or hemorrhage secondary to rapid expansion of a pre-existing pituitary tumor. Diplopia can occur from lateral extension of the sellar lesion to the cavernous sinus with concomitant ocular motor cranial neuropathies or in some cases diplopia might result from the non-paretic retinal hemifield slide phenomena (non-overlapping nasal fields do not allow fusion and breakdown of pre-existing phoria results). Alternating ptosis with variability and fatigue is suggestive of myasthenia gravis rather than a structural compressive lesion.[1,2] Nystagmus is uncommon in suprasellar lesions but see-saw nystagmus has been reported in parasellar lesions whereas downbeat nystagmus is more characteristic of a cervicomedullary lesion (e.g., Chiari malformation).[3,4] Endocrinologic abnormalities can precede the visual symptoms and patients should be queried on endocrine symptoms (e.g., amenorrhea/galactorrhea in young females, changes in ring/shoe/hat size in acromegaly, decreased libido, temperature dysregulation, etc.). Horner syndrome can occur from a lesion anywhere along the ocular sympathetic pathway and although this can occur with sellar lesions extending to the cavernous sinus an isolated painful Horner syndrome is more characteristic of a carotid dissection than a chiasmal tumor.

The solution to Question 2 is C.

Pituitary adenomas are the most common cause of chiasmal lesions in adults, with a prevalence of 75.7 per 100,000. In one series, of these pituitary adenomas, 47% were prolactinomas and 34% were nonfunctioning pituitary adenomas.[5] Other common causes of chiasmal lesions include craniopharyngioma, meningioma, and other chiasmal compressive lesions such as suprasellar aneurysm. Chiasmal glioma and dysgerminoma can present as chiasmal/sellar lesions but are usually seen in children or younger adults. The typical MRI features of pituitary adenoma include T1 hypointensity compared to normal pituitary tissue and slightly hyperintense signal on T2 with variable enhancement after gadolinium contrast. Craniopharyngioma typically shows a cystic and solid heterogeneous mass in the suprasellar space with variable enhancement. Meningioma is an extra-axial, dural-based mass (often with a dural tail), isointense to the brain, and with vigorous, homogeneous contrast enhancement.[6] Usually it is not difficult to differentiate the main suprasellar mass lesions in patients with bitemporal hemianopsia but sometimes the radiographic findings are not specific enough to make a preoperative diagnosis. This is important because the surgical approach might change based upon the presurgical presumed pathology (e.g., pituitary adenoma and transsphenoidal surgery versus craniotomy for meningioma).

The solution to Question 3 is A.

The anatomic relation of the optic chiasm to the pituitary gland is important for understanding the visual field defects that may occur in a suprasellar mass. The body of the chiasm is located directly above the pituitary in 80% of patients, whereas a postfixed (over the dorsum sellae) configuration is seen in 11%, and a prefixed (over the tuberculum) anatomy is seen in 9%.[7]

Because pituitary adenomas typically extend superiorly and compress the body of the chiasm, bitemporal hemianopsia (complete, incomplete, symmetrical, or asymmetrical) is the most common visual field defect and accounts for 67% of the visual field defects in pituitary adenoma. Central scotoma, optic neuropathy, junctional visual field loss (e.g., junctional scotoma and junctional scotoma of Traquair), and homonymous hemianopsia (optic tract) occur with less frequency but may occur (Fig. 16.2). Junctional visual field defects include optic neuropathy in one eye and a contralateral superior temporal defect in the fellow eye (junctional scotoma) and monocular temporal (or nasal) hemianopic visual field loss (junctional scotoma of Traquair).

The solution to Question 4 is B.

As noted above, a junctional scotoma is caused by a lesion at the junction of the optic nerve on one side and the optic chiasm affecting the crossing nasal fibers from the contralateral eye. Lesions may produce an ipsilateral optic nerve involvement that results in an ipsilateral central scotoma or other optic nerve-related visual field defects and a supero-temporal scotoma in the contralateral eye from compression of infranasal fibers from the contralateral eye. In the older literature the crossing nasal fiber was presumed to extend for a short course into the contralateral optic nerve (the so-called Wilbrand knee). Newer work has cast doubt on the anatomic existence of the Wilbrand knee but the localizing significance of the junctional scotoma remains undiminished with or without the actual existence of the knee.

This should be differentiated from the junctional scotoma of Traquair which was described by Traquair in 1927. It describes a unilateral temporal (or nasal) hemianopsia that is a monocular visual field defect caused by damage to either the crossing nasal fibers or uncrossed temporal fibers at the junction of the optic nerve and the chiasm.[8,9] A cecocentral scotoma bilaterally can occur in compressive lesions but is extremely rare. The bilateral and symmetric cecocentral scotoma characterizes disorders with a predilection for the papillomacular bundle (e.g., toxic/nutritional optic neuropathies or Leber hereditary optic neuropathy). A homonymous hemianopsia localizes to the contralateral retrochiasmal pathway. Suprasellar lesions can produce a homonymous hemianopsia from optic tract involvement but the prefixed rather than postfixed chiasmal anatomy is the configuration that predisposes to this visual field defect.

The solution to Question 5 is A.

Several interesting conditions can mimic true bitemporal hemianopsia, including a bilateral enlarged blind spot from peripapillary atrophy, papilledema, the idiopathic big blind spot syndrome, posterior myopic staphyloma, the tilted optic disc syndrome, or nasal sector retinitis pigmentosa[10,11] (Fig. 16.3). In contrast to true bitemporal hemianopsia, these pseudo-bitemporal hemianopic defects do not typically completely respect the vertical midline. Optic nerve head drusen, papilledema, and glaucoma all can produce nerve fiber bundle defects

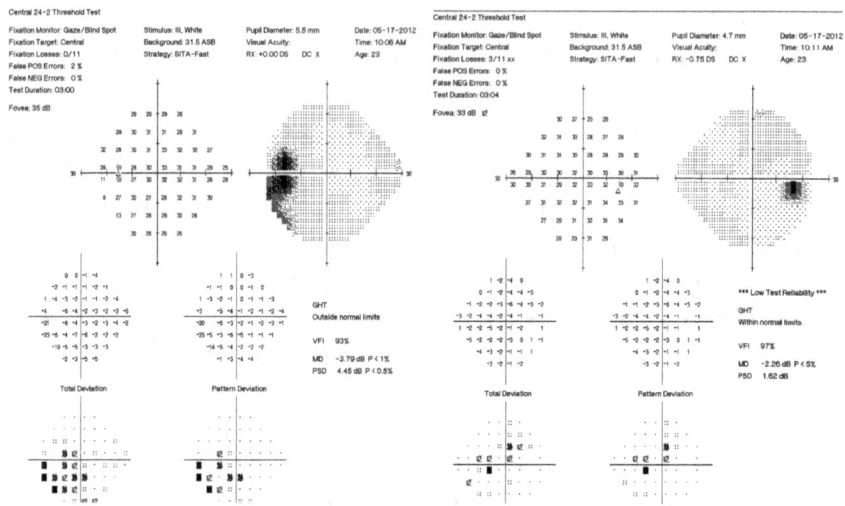

Fig. 16.3. Humphrey visual field 24-2 showing enlarged blind spot mimicking bitemporal hemianopsia.

(e.g., arcuate scotomas and/or nasal step) with preservation (until late) of the central acuity and central visual field (e.g., the papillomacular bundle is spared). Optic neuritis typically produces a central visual field loss (e.g., predilection for the papillomacular bundle) but can produce any nerve fiber layer defect; however, it does not typically cause bitemporal hemianopsia. In contrast, chiasmal neuritis can produce bitemporal hemianopsia that might mimic the presentation of a suprasellar mass lesion.

The solution to Question 6 is D.

MRI of the brain with and without contrast (sella sequence) is the neuroradiologic study of choice for the diagnosis of chiasmal disorders. MRI can also be used to distinguish radiographically between different sellar lesions.[12,13] A CTA is the procedure of choice for third nerve palsy with suspected aneurysm and might detect a suprasellar aneurysm but would not be ideal for detecting non-aneurysmal causes of a chiasmal syndrome (e.g., pituitary adenoma). MRI of the orbit would not sufficiently image the sellar region and the ordering clinician should direct the imaging to the sella in patients with chiasmal symptoms and signs. In addition, meningioma is isointense to the brain on T1- and T2-weighted MRI and without contrast the distinctive radiographic signs of dural-based, homogeneous enhancement might be missed. Like CTA, magnetic resonance angiography (MRA) is useful for the detection of aneurysm and an MRA or CTA might be considered for patients with an initial MRI or CT with radiographic findings suggestive of aneurysm, including a round lesion adjacent to the internal carotid artery with a flow void or evidence for thrombosis within the lesion. This can be a difficult radiographic distinction to make on structural MRI/CT alone and some type of angiographic study may still be necessary in these cases (e.g., CTA, MRA, or catheter angiography). CT scan might be a useful adjunctive study to a sellar MRI in suprasellar lesions because it can show calcification (e.g., meningioma or craniopharyngioma) or hemorrhage (e.g., pituitary apoplexy) better than an MRI. In addition a CT scan might be faster for the initial evaluation of an emergent rather than chronic presentation (e.g., apoplexy).

The solution to Question 7 is C.

Pituitary apoplexy is a clinical syndrome caused by acute hemorrhage or infarction often due to rapid expansion of a pituitary tumor outstripping its blood supply. It is characterized by an acute onset of severe headache, bitemporal hemianopsia, double vision (from ocular motor cranial neuropathy in the cavernous sinus), altered mental status, loss of consciousness, and hormonal dysfunction. Admission to the hospital and emergent corticosteroid replacement might be a life-saving measure for these patients who might have a marked panhypopituitarism.[14] In contrast to pituitary apoplexy (which is an emergency), suprasellar meningioma, craniopharyngioma, and optic chiasmal glioma are all typically slow-growing and benign neoplasms that can be managed with outpatient evaluation and outpatient neurosurgical consultation.

The solution to Question 8 is A. The solution to Question 9 is C.

Transsphenoidal surgery is the typical surgical treatment of choice for a non-secreting, symptomatic pituitary adenoma.[15] Prolactin-secreting pituitary adenomas (i.e., prolactinomas) are a common type of pituitary adenoma and can also be initially treated medically with dopamine agonists (e.g., bromocriptine, cabergoline).[16] Symptomatic pituitary macroadenomas however usually require surgical intervention to decompress the optic apparatus and restore or preserve visual function.[17,18] Serotonin agonists are typically used as antimigraine (e.g., triptans) and antidepressant agents (e.g., buspirone) and are not used for prolactinoma treatment. Cholinergic agonists have been used in Alzheimer disease. Craniotomy is generally not needed for most pituitary adenomas but other suprasellar lesions might require a craniotomy for adequate exposure and resection (e.g., craniopharyngioma, meningioma, aneurysm). Radiation therapy is an adjunctive therapeutic option for non-resectable pituitary lesions (e.g., extensive cavernous sinus involvement), recurrences, or in patients who refuse or cannot tolerate a neurosurgical procedure.[19]

The solution to Question 10 is B.

Up to 94% of patients with a visually symptomatic pituitary adenoma will show stabilization or improvement after surgery. In one series, 25% had complete vision recovery and 50% had useful but incomplete vision recovery.[20–22] Older age, duration of symptoms, and the presence of optic atrophy have some correlation with the post-surgical prognosis[22,23] Optical coherence tomography (OCT) has emerged as a possible adjunctive tool for providing the patient with a visual prognosis for recovery after decompression (Fig. 16.4). A normal OCT typically portends a better prognosis than severe retinal nerve fiber layer loss and optic atrophy.

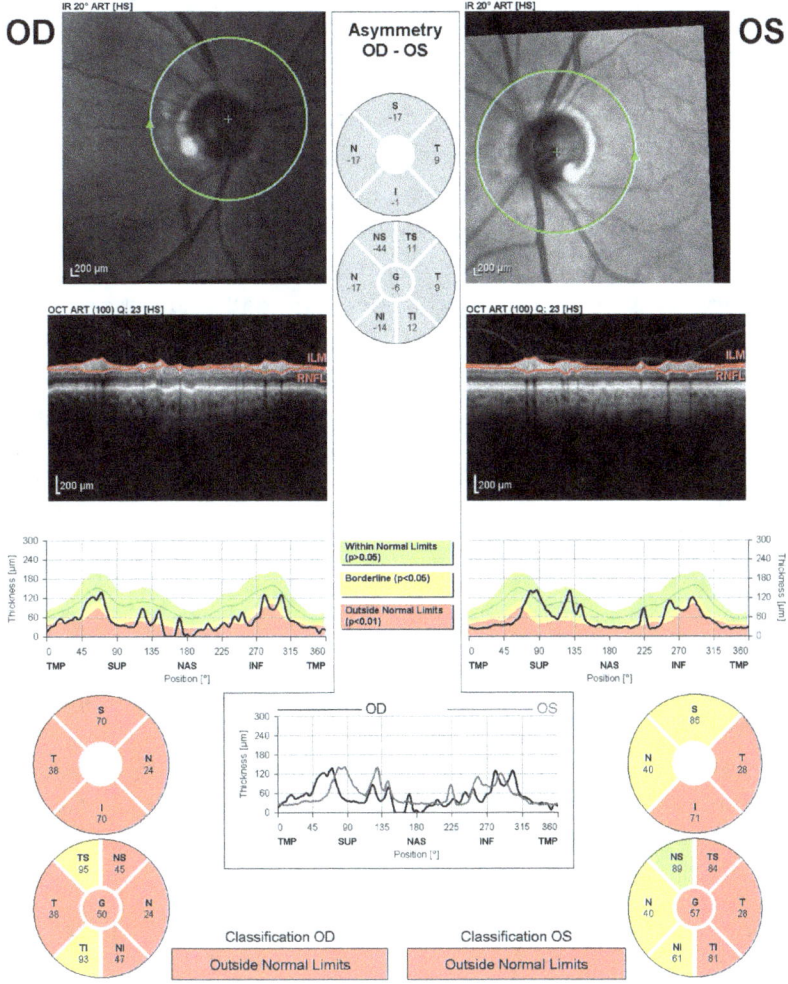

Fig. 16.4. Optical coherence tomography showing optic nerve damage from compressive suprasellar mass.

SUMMARY

Optic chiasmal lesions are often caused by a slowly growing neoplasm, such as a pituitary adenoma, craniopharyngioma, carotid aneurysm, or meningioma. The most common presenting symptom of a benign chiasmal compressive lesion is gradual, painless, progressive vision loss. Bitemporal hemianopsia is the most common visual field defect from chiasmal compression but other patterns of visual loss (optic neuropathy, junctional loss, homonymous hemianopsia) may occur depending on the tumor location and the patient's chiasmal anatomy. MRI of the brain with and without contrast (sella sequence) is the neuro-radiology study of choice for the diagnosis of chiasmal disorders but CT might be an adjunctive study for calcification, hemorrhage or in acute cases (e.g., pituitary apoplexy).

REFERENCES

1. Burde RM, Savino PJ, Trobe JD. (2002) *Clinical Decisions in Neuro-Ophthalmology*, 3rd ed. Mosby, St. Louis, MO.
2. Foroozan R. (2003) Chiasmal syndromes. *Curr Opin Ophthalmol* **14**:325–331.
3. Brazis PW, Masdeu JC, Biller J. (2012) *Localization in Clinical Neurology*, 5th ed. Lippincott Williams & Wilkins, Philadelphia, PA.
4. Miller NR, Newman NJ. (2005) *Walsh and Hoyt's Clinical Neuro-Ophthalmology*, 6th ed. Lippincott Williams & Wilkins, Philadelphia, PA.
5. Gruppetta M, Mercieca C, Vassallo J. (2012) Prevalence and incidence of pituitary adenomas: a population based study in Malta. *Pituitary* (Dec 14) [Epub ahead of print].
6. Lee JH. (2008) *Meningiomas: Diagnosis, Treatment, and Outcome*. Springer, London.
7. Gnjidić Z, Iveković R, Rumboldt Z, *et al.* (2002) Chiasma syndrome in acromegalic patients—correlation of neuroradiologic and neuroophthalmologic findings. *Coll Antropol* **26**:601–608.
8. Lee AG, Brazis PW. (2003) *Clinical Pathways in Neuro-Ophthalmology: An Evidence-Based Approach*. Thieme Medical Pub, New York, NY.
9. Miller NR, Newman NJ. (2005) Topical diagnosis of acquired optic nerve disorders. In: Miller NR, Newman NJ (eds), *Walsh and Hoyt's Clinical Neuro-Ophthalmology*, 6th ed. Lippincott Williams & Wilkins, Baltimore, MD, pp. 228–229.

10 Lee JH, Tobias S, Kwon JT, *et al.* (2006) Wilbrand's knee: does it exist? *Surg Neurol* **66**:11–17.

11 Glaser JS. (1999) *Neuro-Ophthalmology*, 3rd ed. Lippincott Williams & Wilkins, Philadelphia, PA.

12 Larner AJ. (2010) *A Dictionary of Neurological Signs*, 3rd ed. Springer, London.

13 Connor SE, Penney CC. (2003) MRI in the differential diagnosis of a sellar mass. *Clin Radiol* **58**:20–31.

14 Rennert J, Doerfler A. (2007) Imaging of sellar and parasellar lesions. *Clin Neurol Neurosurg* **109**(2):111–124.

15 Lee AG, Brazis PW. (2006) Case studies in neuro-ophthalmology for the neurologist. *Neurol Clin* **24**:331–345.

16 Yadav Y, Sachdev S, Parihar V, *et al.* (2012) Endoscopic endonasal trans-sphenoid surgery of pituitary adenoma. *J Neurosci Rural Pract* **3**:328–337.

17 Maiter D, Primeau V. (2012) 2012 update in the treatment of prolactinomas. *Ann Endocrinol (Paris)* **73**:90–98.

18 Babey M, Sahli R, Vajtai I, *et al.* (2011) Pituitary surgery for small prolactinomas as an alternative to treatment with dopamine agonists. *Pituitary* **14**:222–230.

19 Randall RV, Laws ER Jr, Abboud CF, *et al.* (1983) Transsphenoidal microsurgical treatment of prolactin-producing pituitary adenomas. Results in 100 patients. *Mayo Clin Proc* **58**:108–121.

20 Sullivan LJ, O'Day J, McNeill P. (1991) Visual outcomes of pituitary adenoma surgery. St. Vincent's Hospital 1968–1987. *J Clin Neuroophthalmol* **11**:262–267.

21 Blaauw G, Braakman R, Cuhadar M, *et al.* (1986) Influence of transsphenoidal hypophysectomy on visual deficit due to a pituitary tumour. *Acta Neurochir (Wien)* **83**:79–82.

22 Powell M. (1995) Recovery of vision following transsphenoidal surgery for pituitary adenomas. *Br J Neurosurg* **9**:367–373.

23 Marcus M, Vitale S, Calvert PC, Miller NR. (1991) Visual parameters in patients with pituitary adenoma before and after transsphenoidal surgery. *Aust N Z J Ophthalmol* **19**:111–118.

17

Retrochiasmal Lesions

Nagham Al-Zubidi MD, Pamela C. Carter MD,
Arielle Spitze MD, and Andrew G. Lee MD

CASE

A 66-year-old female complained of hitting the right-side mirror of her car while parking. She also had multiple episodes of acute-onset, bilateral, painless, transient blurred vision lasting for 30 minutes at a time for the past several weeks. She had hypertension and osteoporosis but the rest of her past medical and surgical, social, and family history was non-contributory. On examination, best-corrected visual acuity was 20/20 in the right eye (OD) and 20/25 in the left eye (OS). Extraocular motility, pupil, intraocular pressure measurements, slit lamp biomicroscopy, and dilated funduscopic examinations were all normal in both eyes (OU). Automated (Humphrey) visual field (24-2) testing is shown in Fig. 17.1A. Cranial magnetic resonance imaging (MRI) of the brain is shown in Figs. 17.1B and 17.1C.

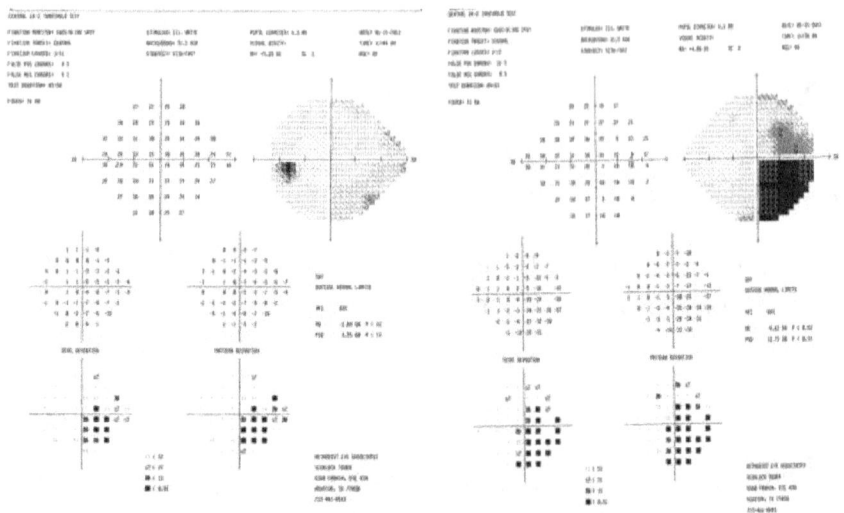

Fig. 17.1. (A) Humphrey visual fields (24-2) showing right incongruous, denser inferiorly, macular-splitting, homonymous hemianopsia.

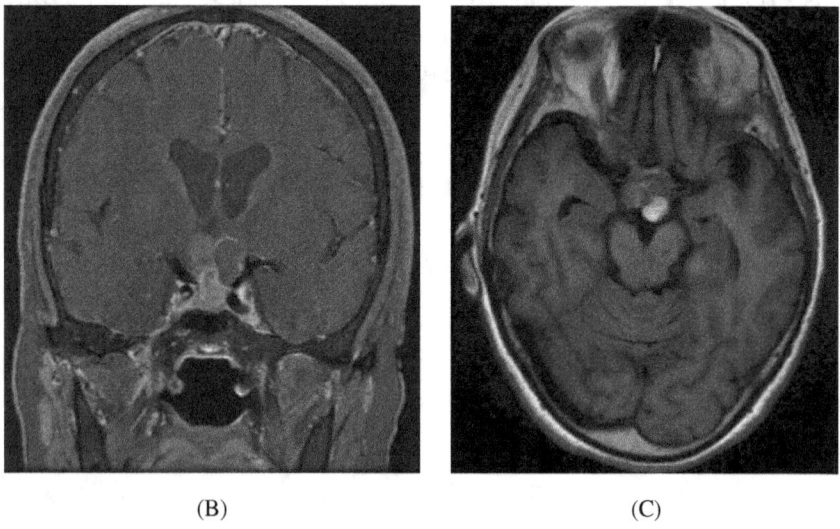

(B)   (C)

Fig. 17.1. (B) MRI of the brain (T1 post-contrast coronal image) showing an enhancing, complex suprasellar and intrasellar mass containing multiple cysts, consistent with craniopharyngioma compressing the optic tract. (C) MRI of the brain (T1 FLAIR pre-contrast axial image) showing a complex suprasellar and intrasellar mass containing multiple cysts that are compressing the left optic tract.

Question 1	Question 2
Which of the following is the most likely presenting finding in a typical patient with an ischemic retrochiasmal lesion?	**Which of the following is the most likely visual field defect in a typical patient with a retrochiasmal lesion?**
A. Painless homonymous visual field loss **B.** Painful unilateral visual field loss **C.** Painless bitemporal visual acuity loss **D.** Painful visual acuity loss	**A.** Bitemporal hemianopsia **B.** Arcuate defect **C.** Central scotoma **D.** Homonymous hemianopsia
Question 3	Question 4
Which of the following is the most likely pupil finding in an isolated left-sided relatively congruous optic tract lesion?	**Which of the following is the most likely lesion localization in a right congruous, denser superiorly, macular-sparing homonymous hemianopsia?**
A. No relative afferent pupillary defect **B.** Relative afferent pupillary defect OD **C.** Relative afferent pupillary defect OS **D.** Light-near dissociation OU	**A.** Left occipital lobe **B.** Left lateral geniculate nucleus **C.** Left parietal lobe **D.** Left temporal lobe

Question 5	Question 6
Which of the following is the best imaging study in the evaluation of unexplained chronic and progressive homonymous hemianopsia for three months?	**Which of the following is the most likely optic nerve finding in a patient with a homonymous hemianopsia from a right optic tract lesion?**
A. Computed tomography (CT) of the orbit **B.** CT angiography of the brain with contrast **C.** Cranial MRI with/without contrast **D.** MRI and magnetic resonance angiography (MRA) of the orbit with contrast	**A.** Bilateral band optic nerve atrophy **B.** Contralateral band optic nerve head atrophy **C.** Ipsilateral band optic nerve head atrophy **D.** Bilateral diffuse optic nerve atrophy
Question 7	Question 8
An ischemic infarct in which of the following arterial distributions would produce a homonymous hemianopsia sparing a wedge to fixation bilaterally?	**Which of the following findings in a complete homonymous hemianopsia would help localize the lesion to the occipital lobe?**
A. Lateral choroidal artery **B.** Posterior communicating artery **C.** Anterior choroidal artery **D.** Middle cerebral artery	**A.** Asymmetric optokinetic nystagmus response **B.** Macular sparing **C.** Unformed visual hallucinations **D.** Seizure with olfactory aura
Question 9	
Which of the following is the most common etiology of an acute, isolated, homonymous hemianopsia in an older adult?	
A. Ischemic **B.** Traumatic **C.** Neoplastic **D.** Demyelinating	

EXPLANATIONS

The solution to Question 1 is A.

The retrochiasmal pathway begins just posterior to the optic chiasm, and from anterior to posterior includes the optic tracts, lateral geniculate nuclei, temporal radiations (Meyer's loop), the parietal radiations, and the occipital lobe. Lesions along the optic pathway posterior to the optic chiasm produce homonymous hemianopic visual field defects that respect the vertical midline.[1] Patients with an acute homonymous hemianopsia typically complain of a problem with their side vision, but the complaint may be more vague (e.g., blurry vision, difficulty reading).[2] Some patients may only complain of visual loss in one eye (typically the eye with the temporal visual field loss) even though homonymous hemianopsias are obviously bilateral defects. In addition, some patients do not even realize that they have a visual field defect and it may be found incidentally.[2] Functional complaints related to the visual field defect may include difficulty reading.[2] For a right homonymous hemianopsia there is often difficulty finding the next word when reading and for left homonymous hemianopsia there may be more difficulty finding the next line while reading.[2] Other complaints include difficulty parking a car or failing the side vision screening portion of a driver's license exam. With temporal visual field loss, drivers or their family may complain that the patient hits the curb or garage or hits the side-mirror.[2] Although retrochiasmal lesions often produce only a contralateral homonymous hemianopsia, other neurologic symptoms or signs may accompany the visual complaint. For example, some patients with a lesion to the occipital lobe may have visual hallucinations (although typical occipital lesions often only produce homonymous hemianopic visual loss), whereas temporal lobe lesions might be characterized by associated agnosia for faces and objects (prosopagnosia) or difficulties with language-related material.[1,2] A patient with a lesion to the non-dominant parietal lobe may also experience contralateral neglect and constructional apraxia.[2] Damage to the dominant parietal lobe can result in Gerstmann syndrome, which includes right-left confusion, difficulty with writing (agraphia), difficulty with mathematics (acalculia), and disorders of language (aphasia). In addition, the ipsilateral parietal lobe provides supranuclear control of smooth pursuit and thus in a patient with a complete homonymous hemianopsia there might be asymmetric impairment of the optokinetic nystagmus (OKN) response, indicating a parietal localization over occipital lobe lesions which would be expected to have a symmetric OKN response.

Visual acuity is spared in retrochiasmal lesions whether the homonymous hemianopsia is macular-sparing or splitting. Thus, patients with retrochiasmal lesions will not complain of decreased visual acuity unless they have another typically unrelated lesion (e.g., cataract, retinopathy, or optic neuropathy) affecting central vision or the retrochiasmal lesion is actually bilateral (juxtaposed homonymous hemianopsias).[2] Patients with ipsilateral carotid occlusive or thrombo-embolic disease might have an ipsilateral unilateral loss of vision from a branch or central retinal artery or ophthalmic artery occlusion and a contralateral homonymous hemianopsia from intracranial hemi-spheric disease. Although ischemic infarction is typically painless, some patients with cerebral stroke causing a homonymous hemiano-psia complain of some pain. In addition, depending on the underlying etiology (e.g., cerebral tumor, brain hemorrhage or edema, arterio-venous malformation) the patient might have headache in association with their homonymous hemianopsia.

The solution to Question 2 is D.

The differentiating perimetric sign of retrochiasmal lesions is a con-tralateral homonymous hemianopsia (Fig. 17.2). At the optic chiasm, fibers from the nasal retina cross over to the contralateral side, while temporal fibers remain on the ipsilateral side creating visual field defects that are on the same side (i.e., homonymous) and respect the vertical meridian (hemianopic).[1]

Homonymous hemianopic visual field defects can be further characterized by their congruity, completeness, and sparing or involvement of the macula or of the monocular temporal crescent. Incomplete homonymous hemianopsias are described by their con-gruity, as either congruous (defect is in the same location in each eye's

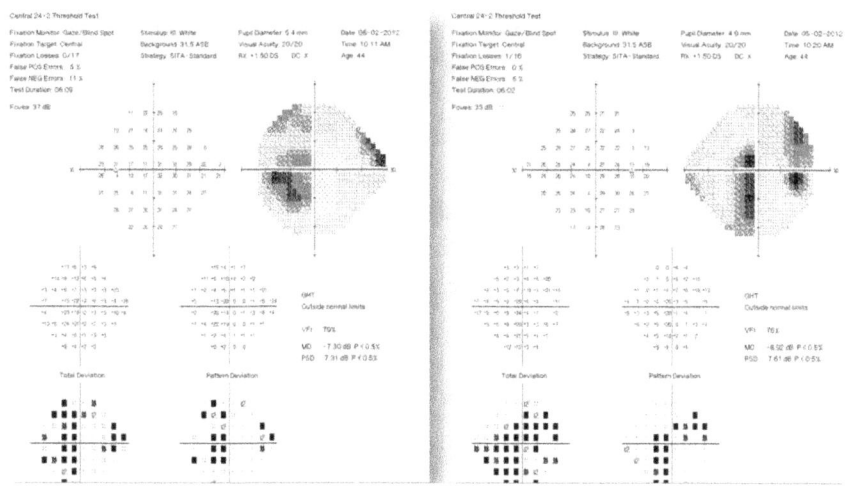

Fig. 17.2. Humphrey visual fields (24-2) showing left incongruous, denser inferiorly, macular-splitting, homonymous hemianopsia.

visual field) or incongruous. As the optic fibers course posteriorly along the visual pathway, they become more organized so that fibers from a similar origination of the retina run in closer and closer proximity to one another.[1,3] In general, the further posterior the lesion (e.g., occipital) along the retrochiasmatic pathway, the more congruous (same on each side) is the hemianopic defect.[1–3] Thus, occipital lobe lesions demonstrate the most congruity and optic tract lesions the least congruity.[1,2] Unfortunately, the specificity of congruity for occipital lobe lesions is not 100% and highly congruous visual field defects can also occur in more anterior retrochiasmal lesions.[1,4]

The solution to Question 3 is B.

In an isolated left-sided optic tract lesion with a right complete homonymous hemianopsia, the right eye (in this example) will typically demonstrate a relative afferent pupillary defect (RAPD). The RAPD however can occur in either eye in optic tract lesions (whichever visual field defect is larger) especially if a concomitant ipsilateral optic neuropathy is present. However, in patients with complete homonymous hemianopic visual field loss, because the temporal visual field is larger than the nasal visual field, the RAPD will be present in the eye with temporal visual field loss.[1,2,5] A left-sided optic tract lesion will damage the temporal retinal fibers from the left eye (representing the nasal visual field) and the nasal retinal fibers from the contralateral right eye (representing the temporal visual field), producing a right-sided homonymous hemianopsia and therefore RAPD in the right eye.

Because the afferent pupillary fibers exit the optic tract anterior to the lateral geniculate nucleus (LGN), lesions of the LGN and any lesion posterior to it, including the optic radiations and the occipital lobe, will not produce an RAPD.

The solution to Question 4 is D.

In the retrochiasmal pathway, damage to the temporal lobe radiations (Meyer's loop) gives a contralateral homonymous hemianopsia that is denser superiorly because these radiations include the more inferior retinal fibers (which correspond to the superior aspect of the visual field).[1,2] The parietal lobe radiations typically produce an incongruous homonymous hemianopsia that is denser inferiorly from superior fiber involvement[1,2] (Fig. 17.2). Occipital lobe lesions depending upon whether the homonymous hemianopsia is denser superiorly or inferiorly can be due to inferior or superior calcarine cortex involvement.

The solution to Question 5 is D.

The imaging study of choice for a homonymous hemianopic visual field defect is an MRI (and MRA of the head and neck if vascular etiologies are suspected) of the brain with and without gadolinium with diffusion-weighted imaging (looking for stroke) (Fig. 17.3). An orbital study is not indicated. Multiple etiologies exist for retrochiasmal lesions including inflammatory, infectious, neoplastic, degenerative, demyelinating, and vascular causes and chronic lesions are more likely to be old ischemic lesions or neoplastic. However, if a patient presents in the setting of acute-onset homonymous visual field defect and an acute ischemic or hemorrhagic stroke is suspected, CT of the

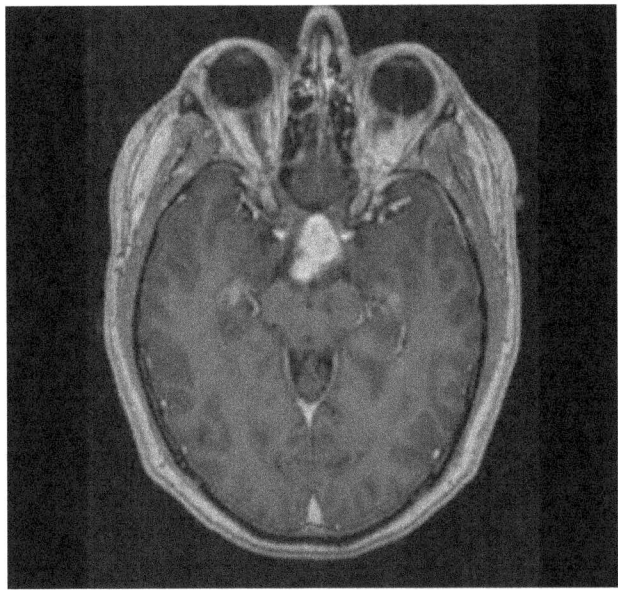

Fig. 17.3. MRI of the brain (T1 post-contrast axial image) showing a WHO grade III glioma that produced a left homonymous hemianopsia from disruption of the right optic tract and optic chiasm.

brain without contrast may be the best first-line study (looking for acute hemorrhage); however, this should be followed by a cranial MRI with and without gadolinium and with diffusion-weighted imaging if the CT scan is negative.

The solution to Question 6 is B.

Patients with a homonymous hemianopsia due to an optic tract lesion might show a special type of optic atrophy (band atrophy) in the eye with nasal fiber loss (i.e., the contralateral eye with temporal visual field loss).[1,2,5] Band (or bow-tie) atrophy is caused by loss of the nasal fibers and produces atrophy that looks like a band across the affected optic disc. This occurs in the eye contralateral to the optic tract lesion because there is damage to the crossed nasal retinal fibers.[1] These nasal retinal fibers inserting into the disc include the nasal portion of the papillomacular bundle, as the center of the eye is the fovea and not the optic disc.[1]

The solution to Question 7 is C.

The lateral geniculate body (LGB), located in the thalamus, is a highly organized structure where retinal fibers synapse along the retrochiasmal optic pathway.[1,2] Lesions to this area are rare,[2] but when present due to vascular insult produce characteristic localizing visual field defects due to the unique blood supply of the LGB.[3] Both the lateral choroidal artery (a branch of the posterior cerebral artery) and the anterior choroidal artery (a branch of the internal carotid artery) supply the LGB.[1,3] With lateral choroidal artery disruption, the patient will have a contralateral homonymous hemianopsia in a wedge-shaped distribution, with sparing of the most superior and inferior aspects of that field.[3] In contrast, with anterior choroidal artery lesions, the patient will have a contralateral homonymous hemianopsia with loss of the upper and lower quadrants and relative sparing of the symmetric inner wedge (termed a quadruple sectoranopia).[1,3]

The solution to Question 8 is C.

Disturbance of the occipital lobe can produce unformed visual hallucinations, such as blotches of color or light.[1,2] These hallucinations typically appear in a homonymous hemianopic distribution, and do not alternate sides (which helps to distinguish them from migraine with aura).[2] Formed visual hallucinations are more well defined, and include hallucinations of people or objects; they typically localize to the temporal lobe. Seizure with olfactory aura also localizes to the temporal lobe.[1] Optokinetic drum asymmetry is associated with a parietal lobe lesion.[1,2] Macular sparing is the classic finding in occipital lesions but is not an absolute rule.

The solution to Question 9 is A.

In most pooled large aggregate studies of homonymous hemianopsia, the most common etiology in adults is stroke.[1,6] Other etiologies however include traumatic brain injury, degenerative disease, infectious, inflammatory, neoplastic, and demyelinating disease.[1,2,6]

SUMMARY

Retrochiasmal lesions typically present with a contralateral homonymous hemianopic visual field loss, and without an additional ocular or bilateral lesion, visual acuity is completely spared. If the lesion is anterior to the lateral geniculate nucleus (i.e., along the optic tract), a relative afferent pupillary defect will be present in the contralateral (or less commonly ipsilateral) eye. MRI of the brain with and without gadolinium is the study of choice for the evaluation of an unexplained homonymous visual field defect, but CT scan without contrast might be superior in the acute setting of possible ischemic or hemorrhagic stroke. Treatment and prognosis depend upon the etiology of the lesion.

REFERENCES

1. Skuta GL, Cantor LB, Weiss JS. (2009) *Basic and Clinical Science Course: Neuro-Ophthalmology*. American Academy of Ophthalmology, San Francisco, CA.
2. Burde RM, Savino PJ, Trobe JD. (2002) *Clinical Decisions in Neuro-Ophthalmology*, 3rd ed. Mosby, St Louis, MO.
3. Luco C, Hoppe A, Scheweitzer M, *et al*. (1992) Visual field defects in vascular lesions of the lateral geniculate body. *J Neurol Neurosurg Psychiatry* **55**:12–15.
4. Kedar S, Zhang X, Lynn MJ, *et al*. (2007) Congruency in homonymous hemianopia. *Am J Ophthalmol* **143**:772–780.
5. Newman SA, Miller NR. (1983) Optic tract syndrome. Neuro-ophthalmologic considerations. *Arch Ophthalmol* **101**:1241–1250.
6. Zhang X, Kedar S, Lynn MJ, *et al*. (2006) Homonymous hemianopias: clinical-anatomic correlations in 904 cases. *Neurology* **66**:906–911.

18

Myasthenia Gravis

Nagham Al-Zubidi MD, Alexander S. Davis MD, Arielle Spitze MD, Sushma Yalamanchili MD, and Andrew G. Lee MD

CASE

An 81-year-old male presented with a six-week history of painless, right-sided ptosis. He denied any diplopia or any other neurological symptoms. His ptosis was variable during the day and was better and worse on different days. Past medical history was significant for hypertension, and he had past ocular history of an epiretinal membrane with decreased visual acuity in the right eye (OD). The remainder of the surgical, social, and family history was unremarkable. On examination, the best-corrected vision was 20/50 in both eyes (OU). Pupils were isocoric in the light and dark and measured 3 mm and 2 mm, respectively. There was no relative afferent pupillary defect (RAPD). Extraocular movements demonstrated an intermittent exotropia of 3 prism-diopters in primary gaze. External exam demonstrated right lid ptosis with dermatochalasis OU (see Fig. 18.1). Marginal reflex distance 1 (MRD1) was zero OD and 4 mm in the left eye (OS) and MRD2 was 5 mm OU, with palpebral fissures of 6 mm OD and 9 mm OS, and lid crease measurements of 8 mm OU. Levator palpebrae superioris function measured 6 mm OD and 11 mm OS. On sustained upgaze there was fatigability and worsening of lid ptosis OD (Fig. 18.2) and bilateral orbicularis weakness. Enhancement of ptosis was noted with elevation of the left eyelid, as well as the Cogan's lid twitch sign. Automated visual field (Humphrey 24-2) was normal OU. Intraocular pressure measurements, slit lamp biomicroscopy and dilated funduscopic examinations were normal except for a moderate nuclear sclerosis OD consistent with 20/50 vision OD, a posterior chamber intraocular lens (PCIOL) OS, and an epiretinal membrane OD. Combined ice test and rest test results are shown in Fig. 18.3.

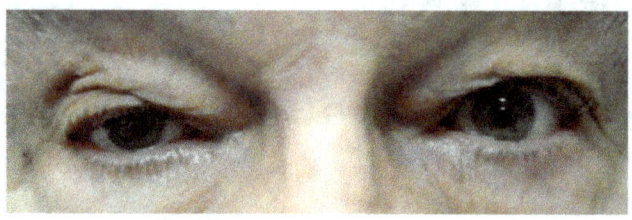

Fig. 18.1.   External exam of patient demonstrating right-sided ptosis.

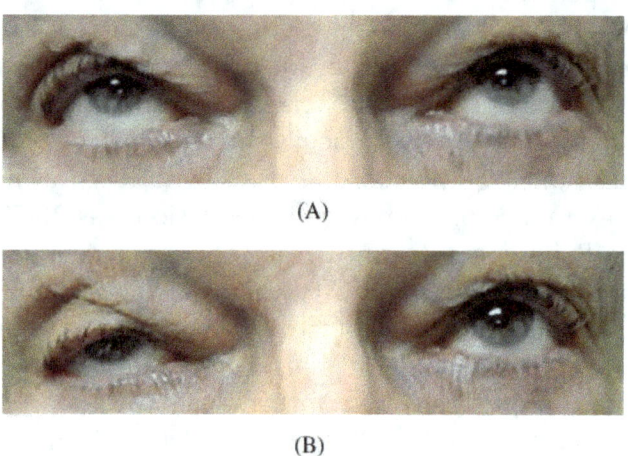

(A)

(B)

Fig. 18.2.   Upgaze fatigability testing, demonstrating lowering of right upper lid over time. (A) Demonstrating right upper lid at time zero of fatigue testing. (B) Demonstrating lowering of right upper lid after 15 seconds due to fatigue.

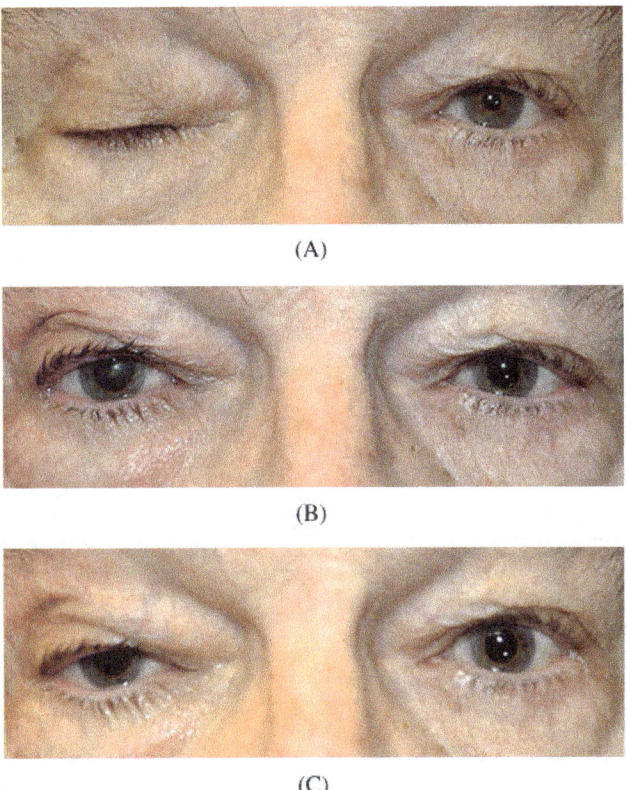

(A)

(B)

(C)

Fig. 18.3. Combined ice and rest testing of ptosis. (A) Pre-test external photo demonstrating patient with right-sided ptosis. (B) Immediately post-test external photo demonstrating resolution of right ptosis. (C) Post-test approximately less than 1 minute, demonstrating recurrence of right ptosis.

Question 1	Question 2
Which of the following findings is most characteristic for myasthenia gravis (MG)–related diplopia?	**Which of the following signs is most distinctive of MG?**
A. Normal pupil **B.** Pain **C.** Lid retraction **D.** Loss of central vision	**A.** Ptosis with miosis **B.** Chronic and progressive, asymptomatic, bilateral symmetric ophthalmoplegia **C.** Fatigable and variable ptosis **D.** Diplopia with paresthesia in V_1 distribution
Question 3	**Question 4**
Which of the following clinical motility findings is most consistent with MG?	**Which of the following diagnostic tests has the highest sensitivity and specificity in ocular MG?**
A. Pseudo-internuclear ophthalmoplegia **B.** Ptosis, miosis, anhidrosis **C.** Pupil-involved third nerve palsy **D.** Complete ophthalmoplegia with RAPD OD	**A.** Edrophonium chloride (Tensilon) test **B.** Ice pack and rest test **C.** Repetitive nerve stimulation/ EMG **D.** Single-fiber EMG
Question 5	**Question 6**
Which of the following laboratory tests would be most likely to be positive in a patient with ocular MG?	**Which of the following imaging studies is the next most appropriate step in a patient with seropositive MG?**
A. Muscle-specific tyrosine kinase (MuSK) Abs **B.** Antibodies to the acetylcholine receptor **C.** Antibodies to aquaporin-4 protein **D.** Antibodies to voltage-gated calcium channels	**A.** Magnetic resonance imaging (MRI) of the brain **B.** Computed tomography (CT) of the chest **C.** Chest radiograph **D.** CT of the head

Question 7	Question 8
Which of the following best approximates the likelihood that ocular MG will become generalized MG within three years of initial diagnosis?	**Which of the following signs is most likely to be present due to an associated additional disorder in a patient with MG?**
A. 5%	A. Hemifacial spasm
B. 15%	B. Anisocoria
C. 50%	C. Lid retraction
D. 95%	D. Paresthesia in V_1

EXPLANATIONS

The solution to Question 1 is A.

Myasthenia gravis is an acquired autoimmune disease affecting the neuromuscular junction and typically presents as an acute, painless diplopia or ptosis involving one or both eyes. MG most commonly affects younger females and older males, with an average age of onset of 28 years in women and 42 years in men. There is an overall higher ratio of females affected to males in MG.[1,2] About 50–70% of patients present initially with ocular manifestations of the disease with up to 40–95%[2-4] of patients presenting with either diplopia or ptosis.[5,6] Of those with ocular symptoms, patients with MG should not have pain, paresthesias, pupil involvement, or loss of vision. Some patients however may complain of blurry vision from diplopia despite the etiology being MG.[5] Thus, MG can present with any pain-less pattern of unilateral or bilateral ophthalmoplegia with or without ptosis. Painless diplopia with involvement of the pupil could suggest a neurogenic etiology (e.g., third nerve palsy) and painful diplopia without involvement of the pupil is more consistent with an inflam-matory, infectious, infiltrative, or neoplastic etiology rather than MG. Painless diplopia with loss of central vision due to an ipsilateral optic neuropathy is suggestive of orbital apex or parasellar structural lesions and does not occur in MG which is a motor neuromuscular junction disorder. Lid retraction is a sign of thyroid eye disease which can occur with MG.

The solution to Question 2 is C.

The most distinctive symptom supporting a diagnosis of MG is painless, pupil-sparing ptosis or ophthalmoplegia with fatigability and variability of symptoms. Typically the patient may describe fatigability as worsening of ocular symptoms such as ptosis or diplopia later in the day or when trying to look at the extremes of gaze over time. The ptosis and ophthalmoplegia may be variable throughout the day, from exam to exam, or even alternate between the two eyes. Ptosis with miosis or any anisocoria for that matter would not be expected in MG because MG does not involve the pupil clinically. The combination of ptosis with miosis is suggestive of Horner syndrome. A chronic and progressive, pupil-spared, bilateral, and symmetric ophthalmoplegia can occur in MG but is more typical of chronic progressive external ophthalmoplegia (CPEO). Patients with CPEO as opposed to MG typically are asymptomatic because of the slow, progressive, and bilaterally symmetric nature of CPEO. Diplopia and ophthalmoplegia with a trigeminal sensory deficit (e.g., paresthesia or numbness in V_1) are suggestive of a structural lesion in the ipsilateral cavernous sinus but MG does not affect sensory nerves and is strictly a disease of the motor neuromuscular junction.

The solution to Question 3 is D.

Any clinical involvement of the pupil is not consistent with a diagnosis of MG, and therefore any anisocoria or an RAPD should raise concerns for another process causing the patient's ocular symptoms or an alternative diagnosis. MG can involve any or all of the extraocular muscles and thus can produce any pattern of ophthalmoplegia including findings suggestive of pupil-spared third, fourth, or sixth cranial nerve palsy, horizontal or vertical gaze palsy, pseudo-internuclear ophthalmoplegia, chronic progressive external ophthalmoplegia, complete unilateral or bilateral ophthalmoplegia, or isolated extraocular muscle palsy (e.g., inferior oblique palsy).[2] Ptosis with intact levator function is often more associated with levator dehiscence rather than MG especially in the setting of a high and indistinct lid crease. Thyroid eye disease (TED) and MG can occur together as both are autoimmune disorders and up to 15% of thyroid patients have MG and up to 5% of MG patients have TED.[7,8] Orbicularis oculi weakness should also be evaluated for in all patients with diplopia suspected of MG as this would argue strongly for MG rather than ocular motor cranial neuropathy.[2] Classically, other clinical exam findings that are associated with MG include Cogan's eyelid twitch (characterized by an overshoot in elevation of the affected eyelid following saccade from sustained downgaze to primary, enhancement of ptosis (an increase in ptosis of the fellow eye with manual elevation of the more affected lid or a reduction in pseudo–lid retraction in the fellow eye), and upgaze fatigue (observed worsening ptosis following sustained upgaze). Pseudo-internuclear ophthalmoplegia with medial rectus weakness is a common finding in MG. Ptosis, miosis, and anhidrosis are signs of Horner syndrome. A pupil-involved third nerve palsy is not due to MG and should be considered to be an aneurysm of the posterior communicating artery until proven otherwise. Complete unilateral ophthalmoplegia with an ipsilateral RAPD is suggestive of an orbital apex lesion and not MG.

The solution to Question 4 is B.

Although there is no 100% diagnostic test for MG there are ancillary clinical tests that include the edrophonium chloride (Tensilon) test, sleep or rest test, and the ice-pack test. In many practices, including ours, the pharmacologic (i.e., edrophonium (Tensilon) and Prostigmin) tests have been supplanted by the sleep/rest and ice-pack tests. These latter tests are easy and quick to perform in the office, do not require cardiac monitoring, and do not have the associated risks of pharmacologic testing (e.g., bradycardia, nausea, GI upset, and hypotension). The sleep/rest test is typically performed by having the patient rest with their eyes closed for 30 minutes with immediate ptosis measurements after the patient opens their eyes. Depending on the series the reported sensitivity is up to 99% and the specificity is as high as 91% for patients with ocular MG versus a sensitivity of 50% and specificity of 97% in patients with generalized MG.[9] The ice-pack test is performed by having the patient rest their eyes and placing an ice-pack over their ptotic eyelid(s) for 2–5 minutes[10] followed by immediate ptosis re-evaluation following removal of the ice. The ice test has a reported sensitivity of 94% and specificity of 97% for ocular MG and a sensitivity of 82% and specificity of 96% in patients with generalized MG.[7] For comparison, the edrophonium test has a sensitivity of 92% for ocular MG versus a sensitivity of 88% for generalized MG with a specificity of 97% for both ocular and generalized MG.[7] Electrophysiologic testing is also helpful in the diagnosis of MG, which includes repetitive nerve stimulation (RNS) and single-fiber electromyography (SFEMG).[11] SFEMG has the highest reported sensitivity (82–99%) and specificity (96%) but is operator dependent, often difficult to obtain, and may be unavailable in some areas.[12,13]

The solution to Question 5 is B.

The serological confirmation of the diagnosis of MG involves the presence of anti-acetylcholine receptor antibodies. The reported sensitivity is relatively low at 44% for ocular MG but up to 96% for generalized MG. In contrast, the specificity of the test is high at up to 97–99% for both ocular and generalized MG.[9] Several types of anti-acetylcholine receptor antibodies are available, including binding, modulating, and blocking antibodies, and patients can be positive for one antibody and negative for one or more of the other antibodies. We typically test for all three antibodies in our patients with MG. Muscle-specific tyrosine kinase antibodies are another serologic test that can be performed for patients seronegative for anti-acetylcholine receptor antibodies; however, it has only been reported to be positive in 40% of these patients.[14–16] We order MuSK antibodies only in patients clinically suspected of harboring MG who are seronegative and the test is generally negative in ocular MG although it can be positive in generalized MG, especially with bulbar involvement. Antibody testing for aquaporin-4 protein is the serologic test for neuromyelitis optica (NMO) and not MG. Antibody testing for voltage-gated calcium channel is the serologic test for the paraneoplastic neurological syndrome

Lambert–Eaton myasthenic syndrome (LEMS). LEMS can mimic MG clinically however and should be considered in patients who are suspected of a paraneoplastic MG.

The solution to Question 6 is B.

In all patients with confirmed clinical diagnosis of MG, a CT of the chest should be performed (or less commonly an MRI of the chest) to rule out the presence of a thymoma.[10] Thymomas, which occur in about 5–20% of patients with MG,[1] affect the prognosis and treatment of patients with MG and probably should be resected as soon as possible. Patients with severe generalized MG may be eligible for thymectomy even without a thymoma. Thymectomy in patients with MG may allow for medication-free remission, reduction in symptoms, decrease in needed medical therapy, but in some cases may be associated with deterioration.[1] A chest radiograph is not sufficient to exclude the diagnosis of a thymoma. Imaging studies of the brain in MG are generally not necessary and will of course be normal in MG but we recommend neuroimaging for patients in whom the diagnosis is not established, for those patients with strictly unilateral disease or in patients with suspected MG but atypical features (e.g., pain, visual loss, paresthesias, proptosis, anisocoria, RAPD).

The solution to Question 7 is C.

Although there are variable results from multiple studies regarding generalization of MG in patients who initially present with ocular symptoms, approximately 50–70% of patients go on to develop generalized MG. Conversely, 30–40% of patients remain strictly ocular MG.[1] Interestingly, 10–30% of patients with ocular MG achieve transient or permanent remission[1] following treatment including thymectomy,[17] with younger age having an improved prognosis.[18] It is of note that patients with purely ocular MG without generalization by two years have a greatly reduced likelihood of developing generalized MG.[2]

The solution to Question 8 is C.

Autoimmune diseases are known to occur together in the same patient. Thus, patients with MG may have other coexisting autoimmune thyroid eye disease (TED), including Hashimoto thyroiditis and Graves disease. Up to 5–10% of patients with MG have concomitant TED and the MG incidence is 0.2% in patients with TED. There are several hypotheses that may explain this association. Familial, genetic, or other immune-mediated predispositions for both MG and TED may increase the risk for both disorders. Alternatively, MG or TED might represent separate diseases with different clinical presentations but with a shared immunological cross-reactivity against epitopes or auto-antigens.[19–21] Hemifacial spasm, anisocoria, and paresthesias in V_1 are not compatible with MG. Alternatively, TED which is associated with MG can produce lid retraction, lid lag, or proptosis.

SUMMARY

MG may present with ptosis with or without ophthalmoplegia and diplopia. MG however does not cause pupil involvement, pain, proptosis, paresthesias, or visual perception loss. Anti-acetylcholine receptor antibodies may be positive and are highly specific for MG but are only 50% sensitive in ocular MG. Testing for other concomitant autoimmune disease including thyroid disease may also be helpful. CT imaging of the chest should be performed to exclude thymoma. Patients with thymoma should have a thymectomy but even patients with generalized MG who do not have a thymoma might benefit from thymectomy. Most patients with ocular MG who develop generalized MG typically do so within the first two years. Symptomatic medical treatment with pyridostigmine (Mestinon) and/or corticosteroids might be helpful but some patients, especially those with potentially life-threatening MG, may require systemic immunosuppression, IVIg, or plasmapheresis.

REFERENCES

1. Elrod RD, Weinberg DA. (2004) Ocular myasthenia gravis. *Ophthalmol Clin North Am* **17**:275–309.
2. March GA Jr, Johnson LN. (1993) Ocular myasthenia gravis. *J Natl Med Assoc* **85**:681–684.
3. Benatar M, Kaminski H. (2012) Medical and surgical treatment for ocular myasthenia. *Cochrane Database Syst Rev* **12**:CD005081.
4. Antonio-Santos AA, Eggenberger ER. (2008) Medical treatment options for ocular myasthenia gravis. *Curr Opin Ophthalmol* **19**:468–478.
5. Grob D, Arsura EL, Brunner NG, Namba T. (1987) The course of myasthenia gravis and therapies affecting outcome. *Ann N Y Acad Sci* **505**:472–499.
6. Gilbert ME, De Sousa EA, Savino PJ. (2007) Ocular myasthenia gravis treatment: the case against prednisone therapy and thymectomy. *Arch Neurol* **64**: 1790–1792.
7. Kiessling WR, Finke R, Kotulla P, Schleusener H. (1982) Circulating TSH-binding inhibiting immunoglobulins in myasthenia gravis. *Acta Endocrinol (Copenh)* **101**:41–46.
8. Pacey SR, Belchetz PE. (1993) Grave's disease associated with ocular myasthenia gravis and thymic cyst. *J R Soc Med* **86**:297–298.
9. Benatar M. (2006) A systematic review of diagnostic studies in myasthenia gravis. *Neuromuscul Disord* **16**:459–467.
10. Jayam Trouth A, Dabi A, Solieman N, *et al.* (2012) Myasthenia gravis: a review. *Autoimmune Dis* **2012**:874680.
11. Juel VC, Massey JM. (2007) Myasthenia gravis. *Orphanet J Rare Dis* **2**:44.
12. Greenberg SA, Amato AA. (2004) *EMG Pearls.* Elsevier Health Sciences, Philadelphia, PA.
13. Benatar M, Hammad M, Doss-Riney H. (2006) Concentric-needle single-fiber electromyography for the diagnosis of myasthenia gravis. *Muscle Nerve* **34**:163–168.
14. Bennett DL, Mills KR, Riordan-Eva P, *et al.* (2006) Anti-MuSK antibodies in a case of ocular myasthenia gravis. *J Neurol Neurosurg Psychiatry* **77**:564–565.
15. Zhou L, McConville J, Chaudhry V, *et al.* (2004) Clinical comparison of muscle-specific tyrosine kinase (MuSK) antibody-positive and -negative myasthenic patients. *Muscle Nerve* **30**:55–60.
16. Vincent A, McConville J, Farrugia ME, Newsom-Davis J. (2004) Seronegative myasthenia gravis. *Semin Neurol* **24**:125–133.
17. Oosterhuis HJ. (1981) Observations of the natural history of myasthenia gravis and the effect of thymectomy. *Ann N Y Acad Sci* **377**:678–690.
18. Bever CT Jr, Aquino AV, Penn AS, *et al.* (1983) Prognosis of ocular myasthenia. *Ann Neurol* **14**:516–519.

19. Marino M, Ricciardi R, Pinchera A, *et al.* (1997) Mild clinical expression of myasthenia gravis associated with auto-immune thyroid diseases. *J Clin Endocrinol Metab* **82**:438–443.
20. Ali AS, Akavaram NR. (1980) Neuromuscular disorders in thyrotoxicosis. *Am Fam Physician* **22**:97–102.
21. Masood I, Yasir M, Aiman A, Kudyar RP. (2009) Autoimmune thyroid disease with myasthenia gravis in a 28-year-old male: a case report. *Cases J* **2**:8766.

19

Nystagmus

Nagham Al-Zubidi MD, Pamela C. Carter MD,
Arielle Spitze MD, and Andrew G. Lee MD

CASE

An 86-year-old woman presented with acute, painless, "crossing out" of the left eye. She denied any other systemic or neurological symptoms. Past medical history was significant for coronary artery disease, hypertension, congestive heart failure, and hypothyroidism. The remainder of her medical, surgical, social, and family history was unremarkable. Best-corrected visual acuity was 20/25 in both eyes (OU). The pupils measured 4 mm in the dark and 2 mm in the light OU, with no relative afferent pupillary defect (RAPD). Extraocular motility exam demonstrated full ocular motility in the right eye (OD) with a bilateral, conjugate upbeat nystagmus in primary position and a dissociated monocular horizontal abducting nystagmus OD with an adduction deficit in the left eyes (OS) on attempted gaze to the right. There was a 40-prism-diopters exotropia (XT) OS in primary gaze. Slit lamp examination, intraocular pressure measurements, and dilated funduscopic exam were normal OU. Magnetic resonance imaging (MRI) of the brain with and without contrast is shown in Fig. 19.1.

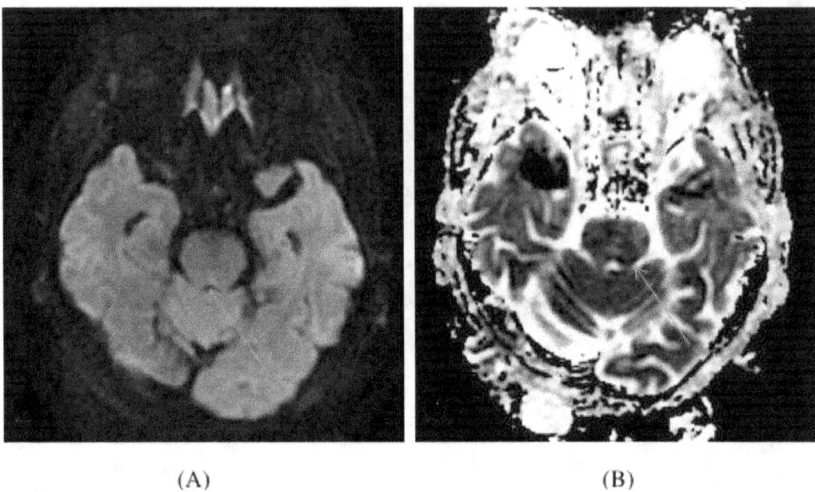

(A)   (B)

Fig. 19.1. MRI of the brain with and without contrast showed multiple diffusion-weighted imaging abnormalities including multiple punctate areas in the posterior cerebral artery territory and a small abnormality in the pons near the medial longitudinal fasciculus (arrows).

Question 1	Question 2
Which of the following features of nystagmus would suggest a pathologic rather than a physiologic nystagmus?	Acute peripheral vestibular nystagmus (PVN) typically exhibits which of the following characteristics?
A. Unsustained in extreme horizontal gaze **B.** Present only in extreme horizontal gaze **C.** Present in primary position **D.** Jerk beating towards gaze direction	**A.** Suppression of nystagmus with fixation **B.** Horizontal nystagmus direction change every 2 minutes **C.** Disconjugate pendular nystagmus **D.** Duration greater than six weeks

Question 3	Question 4
Which of the following is the imaging study of choice for a disconjugate, pendular nystagmus with alternating depression and extorsion of one eye with concomitant elevation and intorsion of the fellow eye?	**Which of the following eye movements is most likely to be seen with a lesion of the medulla or cerebellar vermis?**
A. CT scan of the orbit without contrast B. CT scan of the pons with contrast C. MRI of the occipital cortex with contrast D. MRI of the sellar and parasellar region	A. Dissociated abducting nystagmus B. Vertical pendular oscillations C. Slow phase down, fast phase up D. Fast phase down, slow phase up
Question 5	**Question 6**
Which of the following is the treatment of choice for a horizontal nystagmus that changes direction approximately every 2 minutes?	**Which of the following features is most likely in a congenital compared with acquired nystagmus?**
A. Baclofen B. Gabapentin C. Clonazepam D. Memantine	A. Gaze multiplanar B. Inverted optokinetic response C. Dissociated abducting nystagmus D. Symptomatic oscillopsia present
Question 7	**Question 8**
Hypertrophy of the inferior olivary nucleus after brainstem insult is associated with which of the following abnormal eye movements?	**In a patient with a nystagmus characterized by a slow upward drift and then a rapid downward corrective saccade, which of the following is the most likely location of the lesion?**
A. Downbeat nystagmus B. Oculopalatal myoclonus C. Torsional nystagmus D. Internuclear ophthalmoplegia	A. Pineal gland B. Suprasellar space C. Cervicomedullary junction D. Cerebellar vermis

Question 9	Question 10
Which of the following findings would be the most likely with a lesion of the right medial longitudinal fasciculus (MLF)?	Multivectorial, binocular, conjugate, back-to-back saccade eye movements in a child should prompt workup for which of the following conditions?
A. Left dissociated jerk nystagmus on adduction, with ipsilateral abduction lag B. Left dissociated jerk nystagmus on abduction, with ipsilateral adduction lag C. Right dissociated jerk nystagmus on adduction, with contralateral abduction lag D. Right dissociated jerk nystagmus on abduction, with ipsilateral adduction lag	A. Medulloblastoma B. Nephroblastoma C. Astrocytoma D. Neuroblastoma

EXPLANATIONS

The solution to Question 1 is C.

Nystagmus is a rhythmic oscillation of the eyes that, by definition, has a pathologic slow phase. Nystagmus is named for the corrective fast phase in jerk nystagmus or is termed pendular nystagmus when there is no fast phase.[1,2] For example, jerk beating down is termed downbeat nystagmus. Nystagmus can be either physiologic or pathologic. Typically, physiologic nystagmus is low amplitude, unsustained, symmetric in both eyes, directed horizontally, and only present in extreme horizontal gaze (e.g., right-beating horizontal jerk gaze-evoked nystagmus on right gaze).[1] This is sometimes referred to as end-position or end-gaze nystagmus. It typically dampens rapidly (i.e., is unsustained) and stops when the eyes are brought a few degrees back towards primary. This type of nystagmus is not present in primary position. Other types of physiologic but evoked nystagmus include vestibular nystagmus (induced by head rotation or cold or warm water irrigation of the ear) and optokinetic nystagmus induced by use of the optokinetic drum.[1,3] In contrast, primary-position nystagmus is pathologic and is typically sustained, involuntary, symptomatic if acquired, and constant. The clinician should describe the amplitude, vector, direction, and frequency of the nystagmus as well as performing additional testing to try to narrow the differential diagnosis based upon morphology and the response of the nystagmus to various maneuvers (e.g., effect of fixation, gaze, near reaction, occlusion of either eye, head position).

The solution to Question 2 is A.

Nystagmus can be of central or peripheral origin. In ophthalmology practice, we often do not see the patients with peripheral forms of vestibular nystagmus because these patients typically present to otolaryngology (e.g., neuro-otology). PVN is usually acute in onset and often associated with vertigo, nausea, vomiting, hearing loss, and tinnitus.[1–4] Etiologies of PVN include things that cause dysfunction of the inner ear labyrinth or vestibular nerve (such as benign paroxysmal positional vertigo (BPPV), labyrinthitis, Meniere's disease, trauma, and tumor).[1,4] The nystagmus in PVN is typically a combination of horizontal and torsional components.[2,3] Purely torsional or vertical nystagmus suggests a central rather than peripheral origin. Another typical feature of PVN that helps distinguish it from central causes of nystagmus is suppression of nystagmus with visual fixation.[1–3] Many different modalities can be used to elicit this response, including Frenzel's glasses, video-oculography, or simply using direct ophthalmoscopy and intermittently covering the fellow eye during viewing.[3,5] Other characteristics of PVN include the slow phase towards the side of the lesion, and increased amplitude of the nystagmus with gaze in the direction of the fast phase (Alexander's law).[2,3] The role of the ophthalmologist is to ask the questions that might suggest a peripheral origin (e.g., positional nystagmus, hearing loss, tinnitus) and to refer to ear, nose, and throat (ENT) or neuro-otology for evaluation and treatment for PVN. The treatment acutely is typically supportive but there are also medications such as meclizine or scopolamine to decrease vertigo. Vestibular exercise programs and rehabilitation are helpful in many patients. The Dix–Hallpike maneuver is often helpful in the diagnosis of peripheral nystagmus. If the diagnosis is benign paroxysmal positional vertigo (BPPV), then repositioning maneuvers can be performed by the ENT specialist.[2,4] Depending upon the etiology, PVN symptoms may spontaneously resolve over a few days to weeks; however, resolution may be incomplete requiring further evaluation and treatment by ENT.[1,4,6] Periodic changing of the direction of the nystagmus is characteristic of periodic alternating nystagmus (PAN). Disconjugate nystagmus is not typical in PVN but can be seen in some central forms of nystagmus. Duration of symptoms for greater than six weeks is atypical for acute, acquired PVN that has been treated.

The solution to Question 3 is D.

See-saw nystagmus is characterized by a disconjugate, alternating depression and extorsion of one eye with concomitant elevation and intorsion of the fellow eye.[1–3,6] The oscillations are typically pendular (sinusoidal, with both phases having equal velocity), but can be jerk (slow phase drift followed by fast phase correction). The imaging study of choice is MRI of the brain with and without contrast to assess for structural lesions causing the see-saw nystagmus, the most common of which is a parasellar mass (such as craniopharyngioma).[2] The differential diagnosis of see-saw nystagmus includes parasellar masses, brainstem stroke, trauma, congenital, Arnold–Chiari malformation, vision loss, and demyelination. MRI of the brain is the imaging modality of choice because of its increased soft tissue detail as compared to CT scan. Imaging of the pons, orbit, or occipital cortex is not likely to show the etiologic lesion as well as a dedicated sella sequence on MRI. If the lesion is in the parasellar region, patients with see-saw nystagmus often will have an associated bitemporal hemianopsia.[1,2] Definitive treatment of see-saw nystagmus depends upon the etiology; however, medications such as baclofen, gabapentin, and clonazepam may help to abate the nystagmus.[6,7]

The solution to Question 4 is C.

Upbeat nystagmus typically localizes to the medulla or cerebellar vermis.[1–3,8] Thus, the neuroimaging study (ideally, contrast MRI of the brainstem) should be directed at these locations. As noted above, nystagmus, by convention, is named according to its fast phase; as such, upbeat nystagmus consists of a slow downward drifting of the eyes followed by a correcting fast saccade.[1–3] The differential diagnosis for upbeat nystagmus includes degenerative, metabolic (e.g., Wernicke syndrome), toxic, ischemic, neoplastic, demyelinating lesions affecting the medulla or cerebellum. In accordance with Alexander's law (which states that the amplitude of nystagmus increases when the eyes move in the direction of the fast phase), upbeat nystagmus increases in amplitude with upgaze.[1–3,6] If upbeat nystagmus is symptomatic, pharmacologic therapy with 4-aminopyridine, memantine, baclofen, or benzodiazepines may be attempted to suppress the nystagmus.[6–9] Torsional nystagmus may also be associated with medullary lesions.[2]

Downbeat nystagmus (fast phase down) typically localizes to the cervicomedullary junction. A dissociated horizontal abducting eye nystagmus on horizontal gaze with an adduction lag or deficit in the contralateral eye suggests an internuclear ophthalmoplegia. Binocular vertical pendular eye movements are suggestive of oculopalatal myoclonus which localizes to the Guillain–Mollaret triangle (i.e., red nucleus, inferior olive, and contralateral dentate nucleus).

The solution to Question 5 is A.

Periodic alternating nystagmus (PAN) is a horizontal nystagmus that reliably changes direction approximately every 1–2 minutes.[1–3,6,8] The cycle begins with a jerk phase in one direction, with its amplitude and frequency progressively increasing and then decreasing until the nystagmus stops for a period of seconds. Subsequently, the jerk phase begins in the opposite direction following the same crescendo–decrescendo pattern until the nystagmus stops briefly again; then the cycle repeats itself.[1–3] It is important when evaluating a patient with horizontal nystagmus to watch the patient's eyes for at least 2 minutes to ensure that PAN is not the cause of the horizontal nystagmus.[2] PAN can be congenital or acquired. Acquired forms are typically caused by insults to the nodulus and uvula of the cerebellum.[1–3,6,8] The differential diagnosis of PAN include congenital, Chiari I malformation, ischemia, and demyelination. Although gabapentin, clonazepam, memantine, and other medications have also been used in PAN and other nystagmus forms anecdotally with variable results, baclofen is the best first treatment for PAN.[1–3,6,8]

The solution to Question 6 is B.

Congenital nystagmus typically develops within the first six months of life and may not be present at birth per se.[1] Unlike patients with acquired nystagmus, patients with congenital nystagmus do not experience oscillopsia (the subjective sensation that the environment is moving).[1–3] Visual acuity may be decreased or can be normal (especially at near, where convergence effort might dampen the nystagmus and improve near acuity).[2,3] Typically, congenital nystagmus is a conjugate horizontal nystagmus that demonstrates increased slow phase velocity as the eyes move away from fixation.[1–3] The horizontal direction of the nystagmus remains horizontal even in up- and downgaze (i.e., uniplanar nystagmus). The other nystagmus forms that are gaze uniplanar in addition to congenital nystagmus are PVN and PAN. Multiplanar nystagmus (upbeat in upgaze and right-beating in right gaze) is a feature of acquired gaze-evoked nystagmus. In contrast, a dissociated horizontal nystagmus in the abducting eye in a patient with a contralateral adduction weakness is the characteristic nystagmus seen in internuclear ophthalmoplegia. A unique feature of congenital nystagmus is inversion of the optokinetic response and damping of nystagmus with convergence and eyelid closure. Many cases have a superimposed latent component and the patient might have an anomalous head position to achieve a null point where the nystagmus is least. Congenital sensory nystagmus can be due to visual loss in childhood or may be unassociated with visual loss (congenital motor nystagmus). It may be hereditary, genetic (associated with oculocutaneous albinism and aniridia), or spontaneous.[2,3]

The solution to Question 7 is B.

Oculopalatal myoclonus is an acquired vertical pendular nystagmus that typically presents with a delayed manifestation that appears months after damage to the brainstem (often pontomedullary infarct or hemorrhage) within the Guillain–Mollaret triangle (includes pathways between the red nucleus, ipsilateral inferior olivary nucleus, and contralateral dentate nucleus); it is not an acute manifestation of this insult.[1–3,6] Patients often complain of severe oscillopsia due to the high-amplitude, vertical, pendular nystagmus.[1,10] It may be associated with synchronous contractions of the palate, face, pharynx, and other muscle groups, giving rise to the name "oculopalatal myoclonus"[1–3] (Fig. 19.2). Thus, in any patient with a vertical, pendular nystagmus (i.e., not clearly upbeat or downbeat nystagmus) the key and differentiating feature of oculopalatal myoclonus can be demonstrated by having the patient open their mouth for the clinician to observe the palate (uvula) for abnormal vertical movements. Typical MRI findings include hyperintensity and hypertrophy of the inferior olivary nucleus on T2-weighted images.[1–3,10] In contrast, downbeat nystagmus is associated with a lesion of the cervicomedullary junction[1–3]; purely torsional nystagmus is typically associated with a medullary lesion[2]; and dissociated horizontal abducting nystagmus

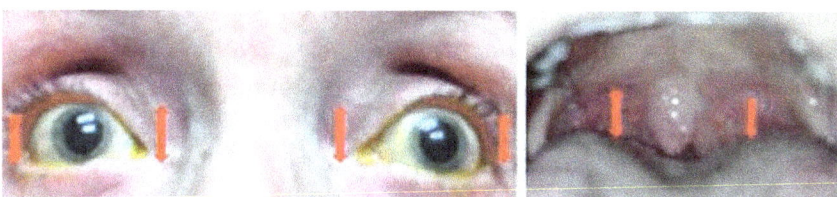

Fig. 19.2. Oculopalatal myoclonus (vertical pendular nystagmus with pendular oscillation of the palate) in an 80-year-old female with pontomedullary hemorrhage.

on contralateral gaze is the hallmark of the internuclear ophthalmoplegia due to a lesion at the medial longitudinal fasciculus.[1,2]

The solution to Question 8 is C.

Downbeat nystagmus, the most common type of central vestibular nystagmus, consists of involuntary, slow upward drifting of the eyes, followed immediately by a fast, downward saccade[1–3,6,8] (Fig. 19.2D). Other types of central vestibular nystagmus include upbeat, torsional, and periodic alternating nystagmus. Downbeat nystagmus is characteristic of disruption to the vestibulocerebellum.[1–3,6] A structural lesion at the cervicomedullary junction, such as Arnold–Chiari Type I malformation, is a common cause of downbeat nystagmus.[1,2,6] Other etiologies include drugs (e.g., alcohol, lithium, anticonvulsants), tumors, nutritional problems (Wernicke syndrome, magnesium deficiency), paraneoplastic syndromes, demyelination, and stroke.[1–3,6,8] An MRI of the brain with contrast is the preferred imaging study for unexplained downbeat nystagmus. Pharmacologic treatment options include 4-aminopyridine, gabapentin, benzodiazepines, memantine, and baclofen.[2,6,8]

Pineal tumors are associated with convergence-retraction nystagmus as part of the dorsal midbrain syndrome.[3] Pituitary adenoma, craniopharyngioma, and other parasellar tumors are associated with see-saw nystagmus.[2]

The solution to Question 9 is B.

Internuclear ophthalmoplegia occurs with a lesion to medial longitudinal fasciculus. It results in a non-sustained, dissociated horizontal abducting nystagmus in the eye contralateral to the MLF lesion during lateral gaze away from the side of the lesion. In a patient with internuclear ophthalmoplegia, there is a concomitant slowing or absence of adduction in the eye ipsilateral to the lesion.[1–3,11] Common causes of insults to the MLF include multiple sclerosis, stroke, and tumors[1–3] (Fig. 19.3).

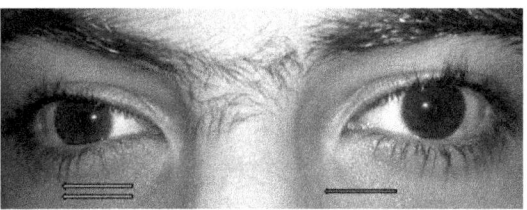

Fig. 19.3. Internuclear ophthalmoplegia (INO) consists of contralateral dissociated jerk nystagmus on abduction with ipsilateral adduction lag.

The solution to Question 10 is D.

Opsoclonus is not technically a form of nystagmus because it lacks a slow phase, but is included in this chapter because it is a clinically important involuntary eye movement. It is a bilateral saccadic intrusion abnormality that is characterized by involuntary, fast (saccadic), multidirectional, conjugate ocular movements.[1,3] It is considered a more severe form of ocular flutter (which is similar in morphology except that in contrast to the multivectorial opsoclonus, ocular flutter only occurs in the horizontal plane).[1] In adults, the most common etiologies for opsoclonus are post-infectious and paraneoplastic.[1] In children, however, paraneoplastic opsoclonus due to neuroblastoma may be present in up to 50% of cases.[1] Nonetheless, only approximately 2% of children with neuroblastoma have opsoclonus.[1] Typically, these patients with opsoclonus have a low-stage neuroblastoma (stage I or II).[1] If neuroblastoma is present, surgical removal of the tumor is recommended. Because the mechanism of opsoclonus in neuroblastoma patients is hypothesized to be paraneoplastic, additional treatment includes intravenous corticosteroids, immunoglobulin, or rituximab.[1,3]

Opsoclonus in children or adults should prompt a neoplastic and paraneoplastic workup, as approximately 20% of adults with opsoclonus have an underlying malignancy (typically small cell lung carcinoma, breast cancer, or ovarian cancer).[1,3,12]

SUMMARY

Pathologic nystagmus is an involuntary rhythmic eye oscillation characterized by a pathologic slow phase component and in jerk nystagmus a fast phase corrective saccade. Symptoms of nystagmus may include oscillopsia (a sensation that the environment is moving) or blurred vision; however, congenital nystagmus lacks oscillopsia. The common localizing forms of nystagmus are upbeat-vermis, downbeat–cervicomedullary junction, convergence-retraction–dorsal midbrain, and see-saw–third ventricular/parasellar region. Other forms of nystagmus have less localizing value, but brainstem structural lesions may be associated with any of these forms of nystagmus. As such, the imaging study of choice for most types of nystagmus is MRI of the brain with and without contrast. For most forms of nystagmus, pharmacologic treatment is not very effective but medications including baclofen, benzodiazepines, gabapentin, and memantine have been tried with variable success. Some patients with a null point can have prism therapy or strabismus surgery to move the null point to primary position.

REFERENCES

1. Burde RM, Savino PJ, Trobe JD. (2002) *Clinical Decisions in Neuro-Ophthalmology*, 3rd ed. Mosby, St Louis, MO.
2. Skuta GL, Cantor LB, Weiss JS. (2009) *Basic and Clinical Science Course: Neuro-Ophthalmology*. American Academy of Ophthalmology, San Francisco, CA.
3. Kline LB, Bajandas FJ. (2008) *Neuro-Ophthalmology Review Manual*, 6th ed. Slack, Thorofare, NJ.
4. Baloh RW. (2003) Clinical practice: vestibular neuritis. *N Engl J Med* **348**: 1027–1032.
5. Hirvonen TP, Juhola M, Aalto H. (2012) Suppression of spontaneous nystagmus during different visual fixation conditions. *Eur Arch Otorhinolaryngol* **269**: 1759–1762.
6. Ehrhardt D, Eggenberger E. (2012) Medical treatment of acquired nystagmus. *Curr Opin Ophthalmol* **23**:510–516.
7. Thurtell MJ, Leigh RJ. (2012) Treatment of nystagmus. *Curr Treat Options Neurol* **14**:60–72.

8. Mehta RA, Kennard C. (2012) The pharmacological treatment of acquired nystagmus. *Pract Neurol* **12**:147–153.

9. Dieterich M, Straube A, Brandt T, *et al.* (1991) The effects of baclofen and cholinergic drugs on upbeat and downbeat nystagmus. *J Neurol Neurosurg Psychiatry* **54**:627–632.

10. Talks SJ, Elston JS. (1997) Oculopalatal myoclonus: eye movement studies, MRI findings and the difficulty of treatment. *Eye (Lond)* **11**:19–24.

11. Zee DS. (1992) Internuclear ophthalmoplegia: pathophysiology and diagnosis. *Baillieres Clin Neurol* **1**:455–470.

12. Rothenberg AB, Berdon WE, D'Angio GJ, *et al.* (2009) The association between neuroblastoma and opsoclonus-myoclonus syndrome: a historical review. *Pediatr Radiol* **39**:723–726.

20

Non-Organic Vision Loss

Nagham Al-Zubidi MD, Bryan Whitlow BS,
Arielle Spitze MD, Sushma Yalamanchili MD,
and Andrew G. Lee MD

CASE

A 22-year-old female presented after she fell and hit her head on the car door, with decreased vision in the right eye (OD). Past medical history was significant for ventriculoperitoneal shunt (VPS) and for pseudotumor cerebri diagnosed several years prior. In addition to the visual loss OD, she complained of four episodes, lasting approximately 1 minute, of shaking in all four extremities, headache, right leg sensory abnormalities, and left eye (OS) pain. The remainder of the past medical, surgical, social, and family history was non-contributory. On examination, the patient was alert and oriented and there was no focal neurological defect. Best-corrected visual acuity was 20/200 OD and 20/20 OS. The pupils measured 5 mm in the dark and 3 mm in the light and there was no relative afferent pupillary defect (RAPD). Extraocular motility, intraocular pressure measurements, anterior segment, and funduscopic exams were normal in both eyes (OU). There was no papilledema or optic atrophy seen OU. Automated and confrontation visual field testing showed a constriction to a 5-degree island OU. Saccade testing showed normal and accurate saccades into the supposedly blind visual field OU. The 5-degree island did not expand (Fig. 20.1) at 1 m and 2 m testing to confrontation OU, consistent with a tunnel visual field. The patient had normal stereoacuity testing at 40 seconds of arc, consistent with 20/20 visual acuity OU. The patient reported seeing two vertically displaced 20/25 Snellen letter "e"s after a four base-down vertical prism was placed over the normal seeing left eye. All of these responses were considered evidence for non-organic overlay. The patient had been admitted to the neurology service. MRI of the brain showed the shunt in good position with no ventriculomegaly. Electroencephalography showed no epileptiform activity but multiple pseudoseizures were noted during testing. A final discharge diagnosis of non-organic overlay was made. The patient was reassured and on follow-up exam six weeks later her vision had returned to normal 20/20 OU.

Question 1	Question 2
Which of the following findings is most likely to be present in a patient with non-organic vision loss (NOVL)?	Which of the following tests would be best for detecting monocular NOVL in a patient claiming 20/20 OD and 20/100 OS?
A. Relative afferent pupillary defect **B.** Optic atrophy **C.** Tunnel visual field **D.** Bitemporal hemianopsia	**A.** Monocular vertical prism test OD **B.** Tangent screen at 1 m and 2 m **C.** Mirror test with right eye closed **D.** Response to visual threat test
Question 3	Question 4
Which of the following responses is organic in a patient claiming 20/100 OD and 20/20 OS and a 4 base-down prism OS?	Which of the following tests is the most useful for binocular NOVL at the 20/80 level OU?
A. Two vertically oriented 20/20 letters **B.** One 20/20 letter **C.** Two vertically oriented 20/100 letters only **D.** One vertical and one horizontal 20/20 letter	**A.** Monocular vertical prism test **B.** Stereoacuity test **C.** Mirror test **D.** Optokinetic stimulus

Question 5	Question 6
Which of the following visual field results OD is most likely to be organic in a patient with a normal visual field OS?	**Which of the following is the best initial management of patients with NOVL?**
A. Tunnel field at 1 m and 2 m testing OD B. Spiraling isopters on Goldmann testing C. Binocular field demonstrates continued presence of monocular hemianopsia OD D. Central scotoma OD	A. Urgent psychiatric admission B. Direct confrontation about malingering C. Reassurance about lack of pathology D. Reporting of non-organic loss to division of motor vehicles and suspension of license
Question 7	**Question 8**
Which of the following is the most common psychiatric disorder in patients with NOVL?	**Which of the following features differentiate malingering from conversion disorder-related NOVL?**
A. Paranoid schizophrenia B. Bipolar affective disorder C. Narcissistic personality disorder D. No consistent psychiatric diagnosis	A. Binocular blindness B. Monocular blindness C. Non-organic test results on exam D. Secondary gain

EXPLANATIONS

The solution to Question 1 is C.

Patients with non-organic vision loss may present with visual acuity and/or visual field loss that may be mild or moderate, unilateral or bilateral, transient or constant. For each of these presentations of NOVL the clinician has several different strategies to confirm that the patient does indeed have a non-organic disorder. The defining features of NOVL are (1) a normal examination without an organic or physiological cause to explain all of the patient's symptoms and (2) proof that the patient can see better than their claimed level of vision.[1] It is often the second requirement that is omitted in patient examinations and it is critical to prove that a patient's condition is non-organic before labeling it as such. In addition, both organic and non-organic disease can occur together (i.e., non-organic overlay) and a careful assessment is needed to ensure that there is no underlying organic cause in such patients.[2] Clinicians should devote additional time and effort to exclude organic and pathologic signs such as an RAPD and optic disc edema or optic atrophy. Many patients with unexplained visual loss choose to have a constricted visual field as their presentation of NOVL. As will be discussed in more detail below, this tunnel field does not expand at 1 m and 2 m testing and remains a constricted tunnel rather than the physiologic funnel expansion of the visual field with increasing target distance. Unfortunately, eye pain (and any subjective symptom) can occur in both organic and non-organic etiologies for visual loss and is not a differentiating feature.

The solution to Question 2 is A. The solution to Question 3 is B.

In a patient with visual acuity loss that is monocular or markedly asymmetric but only in the mild impairment range (e.g., 20/25–20/200) a monocular vertical prism test might be useful. The prism (e.g., 4 base-down) is placed in front of the better seeing eye (in this case OD). When viewing the 20/40 letter and with both eyes open, if the visual loss is organic then the patient should only see one 20/40 letter with the right eye. The 20/100 left eye should not be able to resolve the 20/40 letter. In contrast, in monocular NOVL, when the prism is put over the good right eye the patient will report that there are two vertically displaced 20/40 letters. This proves the claimed 20/100 eye is able to see 20/40. It is critical to explain to the patient that the prism bends the light and that the test is being performed on the good eye (OD) first. The beauty of the monocular prism test is that the patient does not realize that testing of the right eye is actually testing both eyes and that seeing two images is the non-organic response. In addition, if an organic (i.e., a single 20/40 letter seen under binocular viewing) response is given then more aggressive evaluation can be performed to find an organic etiology rather than wasting additional time trying to prove the patient to be non-organic. One study demonstrated that 31 out of 35 people suspected of monocular NOVL reported seeing two images, confirming NOVL. The remaining four patients were later found to have occult organic pathology.[3] Another potentially useful test for NOVL is the duochrome test. In this test the red-green glasses are used so that each eye only sees letters in the complementary color. The Snellen chart can be made to be half red and half green on any individual line and the patient can be tested under monocular or binocular conditions. Unfortunately, the test is easy to defeat because the patient can simply close one or the other eye and thus figure out the appropriate response. Fogging is another commonly used test but has some important disadvantages. Fogging is done by adding lenses of progressively increasing power in front of the good eye after testing the visual acuity in both eyes. This will cause blurring of vision in the good eye which may allow the actual acuity in the affected eye to be determined. Unfortunately, the disadvantage of this test is that it may make the patient suspicious and fail to further cooperate with the test. Using rotating cylinders in the good eye (fogging the normal eye) and rotating spheres in the supposed bad eye as a fogging method may allow a more gradual and less abrupt change in the fogging of the claimed good eye and thus testing the vision of the supposed bad eye. A tangent screen at 1 m and 2 m testing is an excellent test for demonstrating the tunnel constricted visual field of NOVL but is not a good test for monocular central acuity loss. The mirror test involves rotating a large mirror in front of the eyes of a patient with claimed unilateral (with the good eye covered) or bilateral (test with both eyes open) NOVL. Patients with NOVL will have a difficult time avoiding following the image of their own face in the mirror. Unfortunately, if the claimed level of visual loss is better than 20/200 to counting fingers vision, the test is not valid as the patient might still organically be able to see their face in the mirror. The mirror test is thus best for patients with NOVL feigning light perception or no light perception vision. Likewise the response to the visual threat test involves making a threatening hand motion or gesture towards the patient and inducing a blink or withdrawal response. An optokinetic nystagmus (OKN) drum rotating in front of a patient with normal vision will induce a smooth pursuit movement to follow and count the stripes on the OKN drum and then a horizontal jerk nystagmus to bring the eye back to the next stripe. Unfortunately, as with the mirror test this test is only useful for NOVL patients with severe levels of visual loss (light perception or no light perception). In addition patients have to actually view the stripes to ensure appropriate OKN response.

The solution to Question 4 is B.

Although the monocular vertical prism test is useful for unilateral or markedly asymmetric visual loss, the test relies upon the fellow eye as a control and therefore is not a good test for bilateral and symmetric NOVL. Stereopsis testing in this setting is a better method of testing mild binocular NOVL and in general, the visual acuity correlates well with the level of stereoacuity.[3,4] For example, a result of 40 seconds of arc of stereoacuity would be equivalent to 20/20 visual acuity in both eyes.[5,6] Color vision testing using Ishihara plates may also be useful in this setting.[7] Correct identification of all of the Ishihara plates would be less compatible with a presumed optic neuropathy as the cause of the visual loss. As noted previously the OKN and mirror tests only work in patients with severe visual loss (i.e., light perception, or no light perception).

The solution to Question 5 is B.

Unfortunately, producing a non-organic visual field defect has been demonstrated to be relatively easy on automated perimetry (e.g., Humphrey Field Analyzer (HFA)).[8] In addition, the reliability indices even in a non-organic visual field may appear normal.[9] The most common type of visual field defect described in NOVL is a constricted visual field (i.e., tunnel field) (Fig. 20.1), but spiral-shaped fields may also occur. The tunnel visual field does not expand organically (into a funnel) at further test distances (e.g., 1 m and 2 m testing). Testing of saccades into the claimed blind visual field is also a test to prove

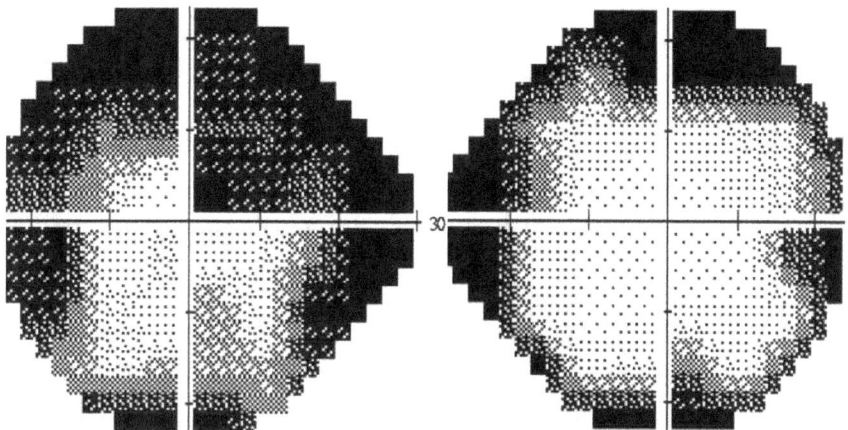

Fig. 20.1. Humphrey visual field (24-2) showing the cloverleaf visual field defect.

NOVL in a patient with a markedly constricted visual field. The patient should be instructed that the test is of ocular motility to avoid suspicion regarding the true nature of the test. The patient is told to make a saccade from primary, when viewing a central target (e.g., the examiner's nose), to a peripheral target (e.g., the examiner's finger or hand) in the supposedly blind field. An accurate saccade directly to the peripheral target is evidence that the visual field constriction is NOVL. The organic response would be for the patient to be unable to make an accurate saccade or to use roving or searching movements to find the peripheral target. Some patients will maintain that they cannot see the target in the periphery and these patients should be reinforced to use their intact center vision to look directly at the target.[10,11] Patients with monocular visual field loss and a normal fellow eye who maintain the monocular visual field defect when tested with both eyes open have NOVL. The visual field of each eye overlaps with the fellow eye and thus persistence of a monocular visual field defect (except for the organic monocular temporal crescent) is evidence of NOVL. In contrast to the tunnel constricted visual field and the spiral field, a central scotoma or bitemporal hemianopsia is a very unusual finding in NOVL and even in the presence of a normal fundus should be considered to be organic until proven otherwise.

The solution to Question 6 is C.

Most series of NOVL have failed to disclose any need for or benefit from urgent psychotropic medications or psychiatric admission. Direct confrontation about malingering is often counterproductive and might incite a negative and even potentially violent response from the patient. Instead, calm reassurance that the examination revealed no pathology and that there were findings suggestive of non-organic disease is usually all that is necessary. Reporting of non-organic loss to the division of motor vehicles and suspension of their license is also an unnecessary and potentially counterproductive response to NOVL. In children, asking both the parents and child individually about life stressors including the potential for abuse is reasonable. Secondary gain (e.g., monetary, disability from work or school, and the sick role) in both children and adults also might create motivations for NOVL.

In fact, the majority of patients with NOVL get better spontaneously within a year after presentation.[4,12] In children, it is important to make sure the parents understand that there is nothing organic causing the vision problems and reinforce the notion that their child should get better. It is also important to make sure they know that they should avoid punishing the child for the NOVL as this response might actually impede recovery.[13] Similarly, in adult patients it is important to give them reassurance that the problem will get better. The most important outcome of reassurance and documented improvement over time of NOVL is ending the cycle of unnecessary and potentially expensive testing.

The solution to Question 7 is D.

Although patients with schizophrenia, bipolar affective disease, and narcissistic personality disorder can all demonstrate NOVL, there is no single consistently present or unifying psychiatric disorder in patients with NOVL and most patients have no underlying initial or final psychiatric diagnosis.[14]

The solution to Question 8 is D.

The distinctive and differentiating feature between a malingerer and conversion disorder is motivation. In the malingerer there is secondary gain that is promoting the NOVL and this is a conscious effort on the part of the patient to deceive. The diagnostic criteria from the Diagnostic and Statistical Manual of Mental Disorders (DSM) IV for conversion disorder are as follows: (A) One or more symptoms affect the voluntary motor (e.g., paralysis) or sensory function (e.g., anesthesia or blindness) that suggest a general medical or neurological condition. (B) Psychological factors are judged to be associated with the symptom and the deficit is preceded by conflicts or other stressors. (C) The symptom or deficit is not intentionally produced or feigned. (D) The symptom or deficit cannot be explained by a general medical condition, or by the direct effects of drugs. (E) These physical complaints result in a social or occupational impairment. (F) These symptoms are not limited to pain or sexual dysfunction. In contrast, the DSM IV criteria for somatization disorder are as follows: (A) A history of many physical symptoms (four sites of pain, two gastrointestinal, one sexual, and one pseudoneurological symptoms). (B) The symptoms begin before the age of 30 years. (C) These symptoms cannot be explained by a known general medical condition or the direct effects of drugs (e.g., a drug of abuse, or medication). (D) These physical complaints result in a social or occupational impairment. (E) The symptoms are not intentionally feigned or produced. In contrast to this last criterion, the essential feature of malingering is an intentional production of false or exaggerated physical or psychological symptoms, motivated by external incentives such as avoiding military duty, avoiding work, obtaining financial compensation, or obtaining drugs. Previously, the terms "hysteria" or "malingering" would be used to describe these patients. However, the term "hysteria" has been stricken from the DSM IV and ICD-10. We prefer the term "non-organic vision loss" as opposed to attempting to make a DSM diagnosis since ophthalmologists are not trained psychiatrists.[15–17] NOVL is a more descriptive, less judgmental term and is preferred in describing these patients as opposed to the older and outdated terms just discussed.[11]

SUMMARY

NOVL is a common presentation to ophthalmologists. The diagnosis of NOVL rests on finding a normal eye exam (or no finding to explain the complaint) and proof that the patient sees better than claimed. Several examination tools can help to diagnosis NOVL, depending on whether the visual loss is in one or both eyes, central or side vision, and the severity of visual loss. We prefer the term NOVL to the outdated term of hysteria.

REFERENCES

1. Suppiej A, Gaspa G, Cappellari A, et al. (2011) The role of visual evoked potentials in the differential diagnosis of functional visual loss and optic neuritis in children. *J Child Neurol* **26**:58–64.
2. Keltner JL, May WN, Johnson CA, Post RB. (1985) The California syndrome. Functional visual complaints with potential economic impact. *Ophthalmology* **92**:427–435.
3. Golnik KC, Lee AG, Eggenberger ER. (2004) The monocular vertical prism dissociation test. *Am J Ophthalmol* **137**:135–137.
4. Toldo I, Pinello L, Suppiej A, et al. (2010) Nonorganic (psychogenic) visual loss in children: a retrospective series. *J Neuroophthalmol* **30**:26–30.
5. Beatty S. (1999) Non-organic visual loss. *Postgrad Med J* **75**:201–207.
6. Levy NS, Glick EB. (1974) Stereoscopic perception and Snellen visual acuity. *Am J Ophthalmol* **78**:722–724.
7. Bourke RD, Gole GA. (1994) Detection of functional visual loss using the Ishihara plates. *Aust N Z J Ophthalmol* **22**:115–118.
8. Thompson JC, Kosmorsky GS, Ellis BD. (1996) Fields of dreamers and dreamed-up fields. *Ophthalmology* **103**:117–125.
9. Smith TJ, Baker RS. (1987) Perimetric findings in functional disorders using automated techniques. *Ophthalmology* **94**:1562–1566.
10. Kline LB, Bajandas FJ. (2001) *Neuro-opthalmology Review Manual*, 5th ed. Slack, Thorofare, NJ.
11. Moore Q, Al-Zubidi N, Yalamanchili S, Lee AG. (2012) Nonorganic visual loss in children. *Int Ophthalmol Clin* **52**:107–123.

12. Bose S, Kupersmith MJ. (1995) Neuro-ophthalmologic presentations of functional visual disorders. *Neurol Clin* **13**:321–339.
13. Clarke WN. (1996) Functional visual loss in children: a common problem with an easy solution. *Can J Ophthalmol* **31**:311–313.
14. Rajsekar K, Rajsekar YL, Chaturvedi SK. (1999) Psycho ophthalmology: the interface between psychiatry and ophthalmology. *Indian J Psychiatry* **41**:186–196.
15. Lessell S. (2011) Nonorganic visual loss: what's in a name? *Am J Ophthalmol* **151**:569–571.
16. Allin M, Streeruwitz A, Curtis V. (2005) Progress in understanding conversion disorder. *Neuropsychiatr Dis Treat* **1**:205–209.
17. American Psychiatric Association. (2000) *Diagnostic and Statistical Manual of Mental Disorders*, 4th ed, text revision (DSM-IV-TR). American Psychiatric Press Inc, Washington, DC.

Index